PSYCHOSOMATIC ASPECTS OF ALLERGY

Other medical books published by Doctor Frazier:

INSECT ALLERGY: Allergic & Toxic Reactions to Insects and Other Arthropods. Authored, 1969.
SURGERY AND THE ALLERGIC PATIENT. Edited, 1971.
ANNUAL REVIEW OF ALLERGY. Edited. This is an annual publication.
DENTISTRY AND THE ALLERGIC PATIENT. Edited, 1973.
PARENTS' GUIDE TO ALLERGY IN CHILDREN. Authored, 1973.
DOCTOR'S GUIDE TO BETTER TENNIS AND HEALTH. Edited, 1974.
COPING WITH FOOD ALLERGY. Authored, 1974.
CURRENT THERAPY OF ALLERGY. Edited, 1974.
SELF ASSESSMENT OF CURRENT KNOWLEDGE IN ALLERGY. Edited, 1976.

GAMES DOCTORS PLAY. Edited, 1973.
MASTERING THE ART OF WINNING TENNIS. Edited, 1975.

PSYCHOSOMATIC ASPECTS OF ALLERGY

CLAUDE A. FRAZIER M.D., P.A.

VNR VAN NOSTRAND REINHOLD COMPANY
NEW YORK CINCINNATI ATLANTA DALLAS SAN FRANCISCO
LONDON TORONTO MELBOURNE

Van Nostrand Reinhold Company Regional Offices:
New York Cincinnati Atlanta Dallas San Francisco

Van Nostrand Reinhold Company International Offices:
London Toronto Melbourne

Library of Congress Catalog Card Number: 76-30816
ISBN: 0-442-21685-8

Manufactured in the United States of America

Published by Van Nostrand Reinhold Company
450 West 33rd Street, New York, N.Y. 10001

Published simultaneously in Canada by Van Nostrand Reinhold Ltd.

15 14 13 12 11 10 9 8 7 6 5 4 3 2 1

Library of Congress Cataloging in Publication Data

Frazier, Claude Albee, 1920-
Psychosomatic aspects of allergy.

Bibliography: p.
1. Allergy–Psychosomatic aspects. I. Title.
[DNLM: 1. Hypersensitivity–Popular works.
2. Psychophysiologic disorders–Popular works. WD300
F84pa]
RC585.F72 1977 616.9'7'08 76-30816
ISBN 0-442-21685-8

To Norman Schellenger,
A gentleman,
A great tennis player,
and most of all,
A good friend.

Preface

I have a cupboard full of drugs and up-to-date techniques for the diagnosis and treatment of allergy, plus the old standby management of the disease by avoidance of that which causes it. But I also try to look at the whole patient, the big picture as it were. The patient is not just one illness, one malfunctioning organ, one allergy; he is mind and body working together in both health and illness, and the one cannot be treated, the other overlooked, without detriment to the sufferer. Holism is the watchword, the concept that the whole is more than the sum of its parts. Thus, disease is more than the sum of specific symptoms, and it is influenced by the whole patient, his mind as well as his body, his emotional as well as his physical state.

This is especially true in allergy, for there is a close relationship between allergy diseases and our emotions. Emotional stress may act as a trigger for physical allergic symptoms, or emotional stress may result because of these physical symptoms. So close is this alliance of emotions and allergy that there was a time when allergic manifestations were considered to be "all in the head." Unfortunately for its victims, allergy is a very real physical disease with physical causes. As with many other diseases, however, allergy is greatly affected by the patient's emotional health. And vice versa—his emotional health is often affected by his allergy. In treating my allergic patients, be they young or old, I must deal with their emotional health as well as with their asthma and their rhinitis, their hives and their eczema, the gastrointestinal distress or headaches that have brought them through my office door.

My purpose here is to discuss coping with the emotional aspects of allergy in a clear manner, comprehensible to the layman. A good bit of what I say in this book may strike the reader as simple common sense. We have always made good use of common sense, especially when we could present it as a "shock of recognition" to our audience.

Common sense for a "sturdy mind in a sturdy body" is the keynote of this book.

Contents

PSYCHOSOMATIC ASPECTS OF ALLERGY

1
"Farewell The Tranquil Mind"
(SHAKESPEARE)

His dark face turning gray with terror, the young Australian aborigine warrior stood as though smitten. Then he began to tremble. Spital collected on his shivering lips and he stared wildly around as though seeking a way to escape. But there was no escape. He knew that he was doomed. He dropped the battle trappings of his manhood and crawled home to his pallet to die. And die he did, even though he was in the prime of life.

Of what?

A fatal wound? Some swift and terrible poison? An overwhelming, fulminating virus?

There wasn't a mark on him. His sturdy body suffered no viral or bacterial invasion. No cancer ate at his vital organs. Yet he died within 48 hours.

I have borrowed this famous example to illustrate the power of the mind and its relationship to death and disease.

Why did the young warrior die? He died because he believed that he would die. He believed that he would die because the tribal medicine man had pointed "the bone" at him in the lethal phallic ritual of cursing. Nor was he the only one to believe. The rest of the tribe also believed that he was doomed; thus, he stood alone, a solitary victim of irresistible power. He had no one to give him hope, for he had been "boned" and he knew that he would die as surely as night follows day. He refused to eat or drink; he simply waited passively, miserably for death. In all probability, his mind imagined he was already dead and, incredible as it may seem, instructed the healthy youthful body to die. We are not certain of just how, but the mind, the nervous system, can bring about functional disturbances of an organ, the heart especially, that can cause sudden death even though organically there is no cause great enough for such disaster. It is difficult to comprehend how the will to live, that powerful force that keeps living things struggling to survive, often even against overwhelming odds, can be overcome by a piece of bone! Or any other taboo or cursing mechanism. Yet, such is the power of suggestion or, if you prefer, belief, whether it be in the powers of darkness and death or of light and life.

Anthropologists, philosophers, psychologists, writers of every stamp, and medical men among others have been fascinated for centuries by the role the mind plays in disease as well as in human behavior. Doctors especially are aware of the power of suggestion. They must be wary that facial expression and even body movements do not convey suggestions of bad news and serious illness. Patients already anxious about the state of their health are as keen as dogs at sniffing out the unspoken. How a doctor does, or does not, look at them, how he sits or moves in his examination, the tone of his voice, what he does not say—all take on meaning, all suggest something to the tense patient.

For example, if I listen to a patient's chest with my stethoscope and appear to take longer than he expects, or if I don't say anything during what must seem forever to him, by the time I am through my examination he is likely to be strung up tight and demanding, "Well, is something wrong, Doc?" Conversely, if, when I've finished the examination, I say, "You're sound as a dollar," or "You came through that with flying colors!" his face will clear and he will literally beam his relief upon me. And if I were to say nothing, if I moved about without a word, putting my instruments away or writing silently on his chart, I am sure that he would slip immediately into a blue funk and imagine every dire possibility that he could. Even a routine physical examination can be fraught with anxiety for the patient!

There is even a regular art to all this. Oddly enough, whether or not the doctor sits higher or lower than the patient during an office visit or consultation has emotional overlay. If the doctor's chair is raised a bit above the patient's, it suggests authority, an authority which, it is hoped, induces the patient to heed the regime or prescription the doctor wishes him to follow. The bedside consultation of a crew of doctors and interns around a hospitalized patient has long been a subject for comedy and cartoon, but it's no joke for the patient to have a bevy of grim-faced physicians bending over him and discussing his various symptoms sotto voce. They may well depart leaving him in shock and certain that the end is in sight!

So, in spite of our sophistication, we dare not smile at superstition or the power of suggestion. We are still, on occasion, our own unwitting victims. Mass hysteria, for instance, did not die at Salem with the hanging of some 20 persons accused of witchcraft by several overstimulated teen-age girls. During the last few years several schools in the South have been visited by a strange malady that passes swiftly through not only much of the student population, but among teachers as well. In one school, symptoms began as a severe itching rash and progressed rapidly to nausea and dizziness. Some 70 youngsters and three adults were treated for this odd ailment at the local hospital. Pollen counts were made and pollution possibilities explored. The sick were carefully examined and all sorts of tests made, but no bugs, no chemicals, no physical causes could be found. In another episode, one girl fainted in a Florida elementary school to set off a wave of illness that had the school authorities searching for gas leaks and worrying about an "Andromeda Strain" type of plague on the loose. In another school recently a number of students were smitten in the cafeteria, falling to the floor as though struck down by some invisible force. They complained of being unable to breathe and they felt certain that they were being gassed.

But children aren't the only ones to fall prey to such strange epidemics. I frequently lecture on insects and skin rashes and I have noticed that as I warm up to my subject, a good part of my audience begins to scratch. Considering that these are, for the most part, my colleagues in medicine, it is apparent that few of us are immune to the power of suggestion. Another example of adult suggestibility is the unprecedented business of APS (Air Pollution Syndrome) or as it is sometimes called, NAPS (Nonspecific Air Pollution Syndrome). This syndrome, by whichever name, can be either an individual matter or also a case of mass involvement. It may begin with a foul odor in the air, or perhaps an oddly colored haze, or simply because a newspaper article noted some facts about air pollution or that the pollution index was somewhat high. In all probability those most affected have been exposed to considerable information about pollution and its hazards—articles, books, TV documentaries, and the like have certainly spread the word these last few years. Thus bombarded people are abnormally receptive. So when something unusual happens—the smell, the haze, the media notice—symptoms and strange feelings spread through the area like a grass fire before a stiff breeze. Heads ache, hearts race, breathing grows labored. Yet organically there is no "real" cause. This is the battle fatigue of modern technology. But even if no specific pollutant threatens at the moment, even if the pollution index remains within "safe" limits, there is often a solid basis for both anger and anxiety. The mind is aware of this. The mind has been educated to the dangers of pollution. Sometimes too well perhaps. Lately the world we have created has become as threatening as the world of natural terrors was for our primitive ancestors. And as it was for them, it is the hidden and the unknown that fills us most with dread. We may not be as anxious about lightning and thunder as they were, but we fear the atom and ourselves.

What do all these strange occurrences have in common? They are examples of abnormal reaction to stimuli, of hysteria (often mass hysteria), of illness spread by the influence of suggestion and nurtured by anxiety and fear. They are examples of the physical being ruled or at least guided by the mental. This is mind over matter, brain over body, and it is a phenomenon that occurs even today with reasonable frequency. However, we would be in error if we tried to separate mind from body and if we attempted a clear distinction of their roles in health and disease. They are so closely intertwined that they cannot really be divorced from each other. The most we can say is that there are times when the mind and emotions may be more responsible for the symptoms of disease than is the body, but since the body is involved, functionally if not organically, then we cannot ignore its role either. For this reason, many physicians follow the concept of "holism." They view their patient as a whole, not just as a specific organ or malfunction, virus or symptom. They attempt to incorporate into this view an understanding of the patient's emotional life as well as of his physical condition.

It is also interesting that some medical men make a distinction between disease and illness. With his kind permission I would like to quote Dr. David Rodgers, former dean of the Johns Hopkins School of Medicine, from both the *American Medical News,* September 23, 1974, and *The Pharos of Alpha Omega Alpha,* October 1974:

> Disease is a biological process that can be understood in scientific terms. It is something that happens to a cell, or to an organ, or an entire organism. An illness, on the other hand, is a human event. It is an alarming series of discomforts, malfunctions, changes in feeling state, and the ability to function that occur in a person.
>
> It is an event in the course of a human life. As such, it is profoundly influenced by the background, lifestyle, and temperament of the individual who is experiencing it, and it is embedded in the trappings of hopes, fears, and responsibilities of that special and unique and particular person. Thus, an illness is ultimately to be understood not in scientific, but in human terms.*

And emotions? How do we define them? An emotion is a strong feeling, a mental state, and it is almost always accompanied by physical (bodily) changes. Emotions are the "drives" that bring about adaption to environmental needs and life changes, that bring gratification for needs instinctive to our being. Emotions are considered to stem from the lower primitive and sensorial part of our brains, in contrast to the higher level of intellect and judgment. And perhaps we should add here that it is the spirit that unifies lower and higher and identifies each one of us as a person, a personality. When either (or both) the emotional or the intellectual areas of the brain go awry, our personality is affected. Oddly enough, it is the emotional level of our brain that plays the greater role in allergy. It is the neurotic person rather than the psychotic (whose intellect suffers derangement), who is most affected by allergy.

While we are defining, perhaps we should attempt a clear understanding also of what we mean by stress. Stress is a force that produces a reaction. It is a stimulus or change to which we must adapt. It can be physical, such as an infection or injury to an organ; it can be chemical, such as exposure to toxic materials; it can be psychological, such as the emotional response of anxiety engendered by potential threat; it can even be pleasure derived from an exhilarating and exciting experience. Technically then, stress can be defined as a life experience that causes physical and mental changes in the individual, a state of internal imbalance. Because we will be interested primarily in the effects of adverse emotional stress on allergy, and for the sake of clarity, I shall henceforth use that term, emotional stress,

*David E. Rogers, "The Doctor Himself Must Become The Treatment," *The Pharos of Alpha Omega Alpha,* October 1974.

to designate emotional distress of one sort or another—depression, anxiety, anger, guilt, feelings of isolation or inadequacy, and so on. We should understand, however, that emotions of pleasurable excitement, exhilaration, competitive striving, and the like produce similar physical changes.

In any case, when our feelings run strong and are prolonged, our bodies undergo specific alterations. When we suffer powerful feelings of grief, hate, fear, love, anger, anxiety, guilt, or depression, actual physical changes occur, sometimes so drastically that our bodies express these emotions with illness. Such disorders are often called psychogenic or psychosomatic. The illnesses usually mentioned in this context are such things as headaches, back problems, ulcers, heart disease. However, some medical researchers are widening the list to include such grim maladies as cancer.

When the witch doctor pointed the bone at the young Australian warrior, he knew that he would cause the victim's death, although he may not have known exactly why the young man would die. In fact, only recently have we been able to understand fairly precisely what physical changes do take place under stress. Even so, some people would say that the young warrior died of starvation since he immediately refused food and drink once the bone had been pointed. Others would point out that removal of the tribe's support was enough to kill him. More accurately, however, his powerful fear strained and exhausted his heart. It developed arrhythmia in all probability, losing its rhythmic beat until it simply quivered. Vital organs then lost blood and oxygen supply and blood pressure dropped.

Death by suggestion no longer happens often in our more sophisticated world, but it can happen. In my native North Carolina recently, a self-proclaimed witch was taken to court accused of causing death by witchcraft. She had predicted that another woman would die on a certain date. Die she did, a prey to fears of her own so powerful that she sought to drown them in alcohol and soothe them with drugs. The combination in large quantities was fatal.

Far more frequently, people express the physical results of intense, prolonged fear and anxiety and other strong emotions with symptoms of illness and/or, it is thought, addiction to drugs and alcohol. For example, in laboratory studies rats subjected to stresses they could not avoid developed peptic ulcers. Other animals subjected repeatedly to stresses they could not second-guess were literally driven to drink.

These experiments, of course, represented stress in the extreme; but there are people who are probably subjected to stresses of equivalent force in their daily life–which may account for rising rates of cardiac disease, ulcers, and drug addiction.

There is nothing new in this view of mind and body, emotional stress and disease. Plato once stated that "all diseases of the body proceed from the mind or soul." And we must understand that emotions themselves are not abnormal, nor are emotional disturbances. We all get carried away upon occasion, and we spend a good part of our lives learning how to control our emotions so that they may not disorder our lives. Not even the happiest, most serene, most contented and well-balanced of individuals is always rational, always pleased with himself and his existence. If there were no valleys, there would be no mountains, and the peaks with their superb views are worth a good bit of stumbling around in shadowed valleys. Life often deals out good reasons for powerful emotional responses; we cannot always avoid grief and guilt, anger and fear, anxiety and depression. Consider, too, how dull life could be if we neither felt nor expressed our feelings.

In a recent book, *The Age of Sensation,* Dr. Herbert Hendin, a practicing psychoanalyst and faculty member of the Columbia University Department of Psychiatry, discussed his findings in a study of a group of nonpatient young college students. He discovered that many young men and women appear to be fleeing from emotional commitment in any form. Apparently afraid to allow themselves the emotional peaks because of fear of possible suffering in the valleys, they attempt to remain "cool" and uninvolved. Dr. Hendin found many of them suffering from such deep-seated depression that only drugs in many cases offered them any relief. There is something grimly tragic about such findings, something immensely forbidding, for this is the image one gets also from *1984*–that of a joyless world of robots who exhibit no passions, no empathy, no compassion, but rather move machinelike through the motions of life.

Passion may lead to pain, but it also leads to joy; and–as so often happens–it is rarely possible to have the one without the other. Without challenge and change most of us would probably sink into lethargy. It is when our emotions have outrun their usefulness, when they are prolonged, intensified, inescapable that they threaten to harm us.

Strangely enough, a good bit of our comprehension of the power and damaging effects of prolonged emotional stress such as anxiety developed during World War II. Like the young aborigine warrior some of the toughest of modern young soldiers were caught up in the web of both emotions and suggestion; but unlike the mind of the aborigine, their minds sought escape in the belief that they were physically ill. For example, paratroupers were an elite group of fighting men. Their courage was not and never will be in question. They knew they were tough. They talked tough and acted as such without faltering before considerable hazards to life and limb. But such a role played constantly in the face of endless danger, coupled with poor nutrition, inadequate sleep, and physical exhaustion, can wear down the strongest and most stable of men. Unable to verbalize their fears and anxieties lest they be considered cowardly, young paratroopers often developed what is called "conversion" physical symptoms, commonly in the form of paralysis of one or both legs. This condition effectively removed them from danger in a "respectable" manner. They were taken out of action not because of cowardice or failure to be a man in combat or even by running away, but because they were "ill" or somehow "injured." And the symptoms of their paralysis were real, so real that the affected limb could be stuck with a pin without a twitch or sign of pain.

Conversion symptoms are not malingering. They are not "put ons," conscious retreats into illness. The malingerer is one who pretends or feigns illness or injury, usually with some conscious purpose or specific gain in mind, such as getting out of work or school, or of receiving compensation from an accident, or to arouse sympathy and to attract attention. If you stuck a pin into his "paralyzed" leg, you would no doubt be rewarded with a kick and a shriek. In my intern days, when we suspected we had a malingerer faking unconsciousness, we would exert a bit of pressure on the upper inner bone structure of the eyelid area. It brought him "to" instantaneously. The malingerer is also familiar to hospital personnel as the fellow who forces himself to swallow quantities of tomato juice so that he may upchuck it in the presence of a doctor or nurse to simulate internal bleeding. All this faking is not real to him as conversion symptoms are to the hysteria patient. The latter is not pretending. He believes his leg is paralyzed. And to all extents and purposes it is. Conversion hysteria (or reaction or response, as it is also sometimes called) is an avoidance or escape from anxiety via the mechanism of physical disability. Often the body system utilized is one the patient can consciously control, although the process itself arises from the unconscious mind. The patient does not consciously wish for paralysis of the leg. Nor does he consciously paralyze it.

There is, incidentally, some difference between the emotions of fear and of anxiety, although the physical changes involved are similar. Anxiety may be a gnawing dread of some unrecognized, even imaginary threat, whereas fear is a response to a recognized, usually immediate hazard to life and limb. Anxiety is longer-lasting, often chronic, while fear is acute and temporary. For instance, fear is what you feel when a huge truck hurtles across the center line of the highway toward you, but it is anxiety that keeps you awake the night before a long trip as you imagine the dangers of the highway. During actual combat, the young paratroopers felt fear; between battles they suffered intense anxiety.

Conversion hysteria can be a great deal less dramatic than wartime examples. Civilian life, too, is rife with unbearable stresses from which the mind seeks escape in "respectable" illnesses. Nor is it difficult to comprehend that it is one thing to decide deliberately "to have a headache" to get out of, say, some anticipated dull social event, but quite another to suffer an incapacitating headache, complete with nausea and vomiting, because of one's anxiety that one will not be able to cope with that coming event. Either way, of course, escape is what we are after.

In the terrible procession of human misery that inches its way in pain and prayer to the Grotto of Lourdes, there are probably a number of individuals suffering from conversion hysteria, people who are escaping with illness of one kind or another unbearable emotional stress they cannot cope with in any other way. They are suffering and they are ill, but they are also "curable," often almost instantaneously so. The "miraculous cures" of Lourdes are indeed those of faith. They are cures of the spirit brought about by the ritual of prayer and by immersion in the holy (and often gruesome) waters of the Baths. Health of mind and body may be restored here, even though such health may have evaded the ministrations of overworked physicians; for the ingredients of faith and of hope that doctors may not have been able to provide along with their drugs may be all that is required to affect a "cure." But the authorities at Lourdes have discovered that there can be a drawback to these seeming miracles. When a manifestly paralyzed man springs from his stretcher to walk again, dozens of hopelessly, organically crippled pilgrims try to struggle to their feet to prove the miracle with their own wracked bodies. When they cannot, they must surely suffer not only the torment of their hopelessness, but also that of doubt in their own faith and spiritual fitness to be chosen. Because of these possibilities, both the medical and ecclesiastical authorities at Lourdes frown upon overly enthusiastic displays of "miracles," of instant "cures."

The question now to be asked is, can the mind, through the power of suggestion, of faith, of hope, as displayed by the pilgrims at Lourdes, actually cure an organically diseased body? Bring a permanent remission to cancer? Restore, at least somewhat, an ailing heart?

Probably no one knows the answer with any certainty, but of all the hundreds of thousands of sick pilgrims who have been immersed, and prayed over, and who have drunk of the healing waters of Lourdes, only some 60 cures have been officially and medically recognized as beyond explanation. Still, we can comprehend that if the power of suggestion can will us to die, it can also, in the garments of faith and hope, bolster our will to live. Certainly we doctors need all the help we can get. In actual fact, medical science recognizes the importance of the will to live, of faith in being healed, in the treatment of illness. Thus, emotions can help the healing process even as they can do harm to the body? Can they cure organic illness? This is the final and intriguing question to be asked of their role in disease, but so far the answer had defied proof. Perhaps all we can say at the moment is that the absence of deleterious emotional stress produces a physical situation that assists the healing process.

We do know that the power of suggestion can be easily employed to provide the patient with a more useful escape than conversion hysteria provides. Doctors have employed this means down the centuries with their use of placebos. Placebo, meaning "I shall please," has occupied a place in medical treatment that only lately has come under fire. Normally a placebo is a pill, although it can be a shot or liquid or any medical treatment procedure (there is something about pills, however, that seems especially to meet the image people have of medical treatment). In actual fact, the placebo is an inert or inactive substance (often sugar or starch) that is prescribed for its psychological effect rather than for its pharmacological properties—which is why its use is under fire in some circles as a medical practice. It intentionally deceives the patient. But endowed with the healing faith of the physician, a faith that is transmitted to the patient, it often acts to soothe or gratify, to take the edge from anxiety, to assure the patient that steps are being taken to help him. It *suggests* a return to health and comfort. I wish not to get involved in the ethical debate that swirls around placebos, but only to demonstrate to the reader how small the step is from the tribal medicine man's charms to the modern physician's little black bag and gleaming treatment room. Let me illustrate with a brief tale the power of the placebo.

There was, residing in a nursing home, one quite small old lady who, after being put to bed each evening, apparently serene, would nevertheless arise at exactly eleven o'clock, without fail, to wander the halls complaining of severe abdominal pain. My colleague who was in charge of her health could find nothing organically wrong to account for such unfailing timed anguish. He decided to try a placebo. Thereafter, when the little old lady arose at eleven she was given a two-colored (she was fond of bright colors) empty gelatin capsule, told gently but firmly that the medicine would help her sleep within minutes, and led back to her room to be tucked in once more. Within 15 minutes, the old lady would be snoring, a satisfied smile on her lips. But let a new nurse on the floor fail to observe this ritual, and the amiable little old lady would turn into a witch, waking other patients with her cries of agony and tormenting the nurse who failed her throughout the night. Or at least until she produced an empty gelatin capsule.

Now it is entirely possible that the little old lady was responding not only to her firm belief in the efficacy of the handsome capsule, but also to the extra attention the second round of being put to bed gave her. Emotionally she may have needed this attention to relieve her anxieties and thus her pain as much as or more than she needed faith in a drug. Anxiety appears more intense at night when we lie in darkness. For the old, the night must have its special fears. Thus, emotional discomfort and the physical discomfort of old bones and joints may join. Faith in the capsule to relieve the physical, plus a little extra attention and concern to relieve the emotional, and our old friend is assuaged. She will sleep.

Incidentally, placebos are also extensively employed in drug testing. In double blind tests, for instance, one group of patients may be given the drug to be evaluated while a control group is given placebos. Neither patients nor doctors assessing the drug are told which is the real thing and which the placebo. In this manner, the possible effects of suggestion are nullified even for the doctors involved in the test, for they are as vulnerable to suggestion as their patients and may be swayed by bias for or against the drug. Thus, the power of suggestion has to be countered even in the laboratory.

There is an antagonistic side to the power of suggestion that can work against medical treatment, surgery especially. Some patients insist upon a negative approach to treatment with such statements as "It won't help." or "Other doctors have tried to help me but nothing does any good." When surgeons are confronted by such feelings of futility, they are wary of operating–and with good reason, for they suspect such a patient of having lost his will to live.

Those of us who have made a career of medicine were made aware of the mind's potency early in the game. Few of us made it through medical school without suffering symptoms of at least one of the many diseases we studied only to find it was actually our fertile imaginations at work. Upper classmen, who had presumably conqured their suggestibility, happily made full use of this phenomenon in their dealings with freshmen. For example, one of the early experiments assigned to new medical students was to collect a 24-hour specimen of their own urine for a thorough study–chemical analysis, microscopic work-up, and the like. A friend of mine, who shall remain nameless, proceeded to examine his specimen with professional interest but with no concern, for he was very much aware of his own near-perfect health. His jaunty mood evaporated, however, when he discovered all kinds of dire things in his urine–marked quantities of sugar, blood, and protein. Convinced that he had become a physical ruin overnight, he sought out the professor in some agitation to show him the doom-laden sample. But instead of packing him off at once to a hospital bed or, at the very least, commiserating with him, the professor only grinned, shrugged, and remarked noncommittally, "It's been spiked."

"Spiked?"

"Sure. Sure. Upperclassman joke. They know how you lads take everything to heart at this stage of the game. Cheer up. You'll live." And the professor patted my friend's still shaking shoulder, adding, "All you have to worry about is your new nickname."

"Nickname?"

"Yup. From now on, you're 'Sweet Pea'!"

And so he was.

There is another classic scenario along these lines that often makes the rounds of college campuses and army camps. To me, it's on the cruel side, but it does, nevertheless, illustrate mind over matter. A professor (army officer) announces that there will be an important, nay, vital examination on the morrow which will determine the student's (soldier's) future. After the test is over, he calls in the students (soldiers) one by one to announce the results privately. When the victim, tense with suspense, approaches the desk, the professor (officer) deliberately makes him stand there while he pretends to read or correct papers. Finally he looks up. He stares sternly at the by now quivering student, rises slowly, walks around his desk to confront the apprehensive victim. Suddenly, in a loud voice, he exclaims "You!" and touches the victim on the forehead and, hopefully, catches him as he faints.

Can this be?

Well, let's just say that the story has been around for a long time.

Surely, the reader has had his own clear experiences with the power of suggestion. For instance, many of us have jubilantly tackled an obstacle—a fence or rock wall, for example—intending to hurdle it lithely, the very epitome of grace. Suddenly, however, a thought intrudes: What if I were to fall? And fall one does, victim of the doubtful mind.

Every champion tennis player I have talked to in my own more modest pursuit of the game has said that he knew that he was going to win before he went out on the court, for if he thought otherwise, he was sure to lose. Positive thinking, or no use to go out there! Tennis players often say, too, that they "see" themselves hitting a ball, returning a serve or the like, and their bodies automatically follow through just as the play was visualized.

So, with these examples before us and the prospect of many others waiting in the wings, let us admit that the young aborigine warrior who crept home to die because he had been "boned" is not a total freak even to our sophisticated view. Nor can the importance of faith and hope be overestimated in the treatment of disease. We shamans know this all too well.

2

The Anxious Mind and Disease

George W. was referred to me by his family physician because of severe, migrainelike headaches for which no specific cause could be found.

"Dr. Smith thinks that I may be allergic to something," George exclaimed. "If I am, it certainly came on suddenly!"

He was a well set-up man in his early thirties with all the appearances of enjoying excellent health. I did notice two things about him during the initial interview—his voice, low and without much expression, seemed to indicate an odd lack of energy, and he appeared noticeably preoccupied, as if his thoughts were a good distance away from the state of his health and my questions. Several times he visibly had to bring his attention back to the matter in hand.

The first step we allergists take is to obtain a history of the patient—his symptoms, past illnesses, past problems, plus the illnesses that have appeared in his family. This procedure, often somewhat lengthy, is a vital diagnostic tool. We may ask odd questions, such as: Are the symptoms seasonal or all year round? When and where do they appear? Can the patient associate any special activity or environmental factor with his problem? Does he dislike certain foods? Or is he inordinately fond of others? Does he remember if he had colic as a baby? Eczema? And we ask about his family, whether anyone else has suffered allergy, for allergy tendency appears to be an inherited vulnerability as far as we now know. If there is a history of allergy in one side of the family, the individual has about a 50 percent chance of suffering from an allergy to something himself. If it runs in both sides, his chances of inheriting the tendency rise to 75 percent.

In George's case, there was a history of allergy on his mother's side. His grandmother and an aunt had suffered from hay fever. As far as his own health went, it was excellent. He rarely had colds. The last one he remembered had been at least three years ago. No, he rarely suffered from indigestion. No, he took no drugs with the exception of an occasional aspirin. Of course, lately, since his headaches had begun, he'd used quite a bit of the stuff.

"I tell you, Doctor, I've always been as healthy as a horse. Until now. I've got to get rid of these blasted headaches. They're messing me up at the office, but worst of all, they make it hard for me to help Ellen and she needs me so. I can't be sick! I just can't."

There was real despair in his voice now and a note of hopelessness.

"Your wife . . . ? She's ill?"

"Yes. We found out–oh, several months ago. She had surgery, radical surgery. It was malignant. She's very upset, you see. We don't really know yet . . . the outcome. I have to help her all I can. Try to bolster her hope . . . ."

"Several months ago? And your headaches? They began around then?"

"Yes. About then."

After the usual tests–skin tests, lab work-ups, and a thorough physical examination–I did find that George W. *was* allergic to some inhalant allergens (dust, molds, feathers). I instructed him on avoidance measures so that he could keep at least his home environment reasonably free of these allergenic factors. And I prescribed medication to mitigate his symptoms when avoidance measures were impossible. Finally, I explained carefully the role his distress over his wife's illness was playing in his allergic symptoms and that it was probable that no "cure" could be guaranteed as long as he continued to suffer such severe emotional stress. And so it was.

How then did George W.'s grief and anxiety about his wife's probable terminal illness precipitate his headaches? How can the emotionally stressed mind bring about allergy or any other illness of the body? The how exactly is not thoroughly understood at present. Nor is it possible as yet to designate or specify an emotional cause for a physical response, so closely interwoven are mind and body. The problem is somewhat akin to following a single thread through the intricate pattern of a huge and beautifully tapestry. Whatever distinctions we make trying to separate that thread are done to clarify its role; yet since it is part of a whole, it cannot stand alone and be meaningful. Emotions may precipitate disease and disease may precipitate emotions, but which comes first remains an unknown quantity. For our purposes, it really doesn't matter. When you have a tiger by the tail, how you got in such a situation is far less important than how you are going to get out of it. Thus, we will not say that George W. suffered allergy symptoms because of emotional stress. Or that he suffered emotional stress because of his allergy symptoms. What we will say is that his emotional stress played an important role in his allergy but did not cause it. There are so many other factors that may also have played a role—pollution, occupational exposure, infection—that the thread, the cause, cannot stand alone. This is the essence of holism—a concept that the whole is greater than its parts, that a patient must be viewed as an entity rather than as a single diseased organ or body system.

We said earlier that stress is generally defined as the response of mind and body to adverse stimuli. Such a response can be as simple as crying "Ouch!" and snatching one's hand away from a hot stove or as complex as the grief and guilt that may follow the loss of a loved one. There is a distinction in the two examples above since the first is physiological and the second psychological. It is the second that we are dealing with here, and within the term emotional stress we are incorporating such feelings as frustration, anxiety, hostility, conflict. We are harried and pummeled throughout our lifetime not only by the stresses of our environment but also by the stresses of our experiences. And, of course, no two of us live life alike or arrive with exactly the same equipment to meet its ups and downs; thus, no two of us are shaped or squeezed or stricken or respond in the same manner to the stresses of our existence. For example, a physician in charge of a hospital ward full of patients suffering a comparable disease or injury will find that the experience of suffering that disease or injury is different for each one of his patients; each sees his problem in a different light and faces it with emotions of varying intensity. Thus, the ward physician cannot predict with any certainty how each patient will react to his illness or injury.

How the patient reacts is his adaption to stress imposed by his illness, both the physical and the emotional stress it engenders for him as an individual. His way of coping with his present problem may be quite different from that of the patient in the next bed.

Both physical and emotional stress bring about bodily changes. Stress of whatever origin can alter body chemistry and organ function, but we possess a built-in force that attempts to restore us to a state of equilibrium, a state called homeostasis. Ordinarily, while stress may unsettle or disturb us physically and/or emotionally, in good health we usually can return to an efficient state of homeostasis without too much difficulty.

Now let us return to emotional stress and stay with it. When such stress is prolonged, intensified, and inescapable, bodily changes occur that can do a great deal of harm. Anxiety, for example, can change the rate of our heartbeat, alter blood pressure, release hormones in prodigions quantity, even alter the temperature of our skin. The physical mechanism of the fright-fight-flight response, for instance, has been well researched in the laboratory. It involves a complex sequence of events regulated by the hypothalamus, which lies near the base of our brains and which is the commander-in-chief of our autonomic (involuntary) nervous system. This is the system that guides our involuntary or automatic bodily functions–blood pressure, heartbeat, body temperature, the action of the gastrointestinal system, and even the production of saliva in the mouth. It is the command post of our ability to remain in homeostasis.

However, when we speak of homeostasis (meaning "steady state"), we are not talking about a rigid, static state, but rather of a relatively constant one. Thus, blood pressure, body temperature, heart rate may fluctuate, but in homeostasis they stay within so-called normal bounds as the body adapts to various internal and external changes.

The section of the brain that harbors the control mechanism of the involuntary nervous system and our emotions, feelings, sensations, perceptions, and the like works hard at maintaining our equilibrium with the world outside and with our own inner life. Ordinarily we don't pay much attention to this part of our works as long as it ticks away as it is supposed to do. But when the system goes awry, we suddenly become very much aware of our physical selves. It is as though a hidden part of ourselves has come awake abruptly with a cry of alarm.

To understand how the brain maintains homeostasis, we should note that the autonomic nervous system is composed of two opposing divisions–the sympathetic and the parasympathetic. The former system adapts or moves the body to respond to stimuli, while the latter returns the body to equilibrium or the earlier state. Thus, the sympathetic system ordinarily causes constriction of blood vessels and smooth muscles and increases glandular secretions, whereas the parasympathetic system expands and relaxes blood vessels and the smooth or involuntary muscles. While the two systems oppose each other in their mechanisms, they are both under the command of the hypothalamus. It is the sympathetic system that readies us for fight or flight when we experience fright. It does so when the "intellectual" part of our brain, the cortex, perceives danger, recognizes it as such, and signals alarm to the hypothalamus, which in turn signals the sympathetic nervous system, which stimulates the release of hormones, especially adrenalin and noradrenalin, both exceedingly potent in our emotional life. The hypothalamus also signals the pituitary gland, the mighty "peanut" of our glandular system, to stimulate the cortex of the adrenal glands to release the steroids (additional hormones). Thus fright releases a veritable shower of hormones throughout a good part of the body to ready it for action, either for the struggle for survival or for flight from threat of attack. This release, for example, causes the blood vessels of the skin and gastrointestinal tract to constrict, returning blood to the heart and raising blood pressure, which in turn sends more blood to the muscles to support them for instant action, be it to hit out at the attacking threat or to move the feet speedily in the opposite direction. Hormones also stimulate the heart to beat faster and the lungs to breathe more rapidly to supply more oxygen to the blood and thus to the cells of the muscles involved in fight or flight. The liver, too, is stimulated to release more sugar into the bloodstream to give these muscles increased energy. Even the pupils of our eyes are dilated as though to help us perceive our danger and/or our route of escape. In this fashion our bodies are readied by the commander-in-chief up there in our brains as the emotion of fright is registered. And all of this almost simultaneously!

It is interesting that we also exhibit some ancient holdovers from our animal heritage. Our skin contracts, raising "gooseflesh," which, if we were still hairy, would raise the hair of our bodies to make us look larger to the attacker or whatever threatened. The "butterflies" or sinking sensation we feel at the pit of our stomachs was designed by nature to make us lose all thought of food so that blood need not be diverted from muscles to stomach. Even the "dry mouth" of fear was designed as a measure to counter the desire to eat. In wartime especially, men under the terrible stress of fear often suffer abrupt diarrhea, a mechanism nature intended as a way of lightening the load of an animal fleeing a predator. Those of us who elect to stand and fight (or have no alternative) often resemble the proverbial "cornered rat" that keeps up a constant barrage of furious chittering and snarling, bares its teeth, rises to its full height, bristles, and so on. The pattern of fright-flight-fight is far more ancient than we are.

It is important to note that this same general reaction or coping mechanism to stimuli or stress, this same general chemical or hormonal shower and altered body machinery, as it were, occurs not only in fright but under the impetus of other powerful emotions such as anger and anxiety, guilt and hate, grief and frustration. When such emotions are often repeated, become chronic, the body is treated to a constant repetition of these hormonal showers and remains more or less out of kilter as a result. The individual becomes more or less out of homeostasis or at least a satisfactory homeostasis. The body is actually overdriven by its reactions to emotional stress and something has to give. What gives seems to depend in great part upon what particular hereditary weakness or vulnerability the individual carries in his genes, or what sort of prior injury to his body may have occurred, such as an acute infection or infectious disease. Thus, the factors of emotional stress plus genetic predisposition and/or prior injury may work together to produce illness. We do not really know yet, but the theory of genetic predisposition and/or prior injury serves to explain somewhat why some individuals can withstand a great deal of emotional stress (just as some can withstand a great deal of physical stress—heat, cold, hunger) without illness, and also why some individuals respond to emotional stress with one type of illness, say gastrointestinal problems, while others will respond with completely different body disturbances, such as cardiac problems. When we narrow this theory down to the field of allergy, we find, for instance, that some individuals respond to the emotional stress factor in their illness with, say, asthma, while others will respond with eczema. The allergen that may be the prime cause for both types of symptoms or body systems affected can be the same—perhaps chocolate or eggs, for example. The tendency to either asthma or eczema exists. Emotional stress may be a factor in precipitating symptoms.

Some types of illness, of course, are ruled out of the emotional stress theory, or if you prefer, the psychosomatic picture: poisoning by toxic substances, for instance, or sickle cell anemia, or diseases caused by occupational exposures to such things as vinyl chloride, now indicted in a rare liver cancer. Yet, even in such illnesses, some doctors believe that the level of damage may be influenced in some way or to some degree by the patient's emotional state, and that the psychosomatic approach is still valid.

Individual susceptibilities plus individual life experiences, especially those of early childhood, determine in good part how we respond to emotional stress. This is not to say that we are set rigidly as in cement for all our lives. We can change and sometimes we must to survive. But, as an example, you may be the Rock of Gibraltar, taking loss of your job, illness of your wife, drug problems among your children in stride. You may respond by immediately setting out to find another job, by seeking to find ways to help your ailing wife, and by seeing to it that your children understand the hazards of drugs and forswear them before damage is done. I, on the other hand, faced with problems perhaps not nearly as severe as yours, may take to my bed with an ulcer, or become hypertensive, or suffer from asthma, depending perhaps upon the vulnerability inherited from my forebears or upon the damage of an earlier disease, such as measles suffered in my childhood. We will have made our separate adaptions to emotional stress, you and I. Yours was successful; mine, self-destructive. You relieved tension with action; I tried with passivity. You were flexible and self-sufficient, able to change with changing circumstances and to learn from experience. Your behavior was rewarding in the end. At least, I hope so. I, on the other hand, was too rigid, my adaption regressive. I had not learned by experience how to tackle my problems actively, how to change under stressful conditions. I will have been overwhelmed by life's pain. This is not to say that you will not have suffered greatly from emotional distress. You will have, but you will have employed outgoing, aggressive behavior to escape that distress; while I will have employed negative behavior in an attempt to escape through illness, for my illness will solve nothing. In fact, the opposite is true—it can only complicate my problems. As George W.'s headaches complicated his.

This also does not mean that I cannot be helped. Given insight into my maladaption, given support and reassurance, I can, in all probability, find my own way back to an efficient and healthy homeostasis. I can learn to enjoy positive coping mechanisms rather than negative, as we shall see later in the book.

We are aware these days that some people may be so without hope, feel so helpless about their lives that they not only consciously contemplate suicide, but may also unconsciously court self-destruction in accident and disease. For instance, in a study conducted in England some time ago, researchers discovered that during the first six months following the deaths of their wives, the mortality rate for a group of middle-aged and over widowers was some 40 percent higher than for other men their age.

In a more recent study of football players, the players were asked to record the life changes they had undergone during the year preceding the opening of football season. They were then rated on the probably risk of injury they might suffer in the coming season. Only about 9 percent in the low-risk group were injured, whereas some 25 percent in the medium-risk and 50 percent in the high-risk group were hurt.

A descending scale called the Social Readjustment Rating Scale has been developed to estimate the impact of various life changes upon the individual. The scale begins with the event that can cause the greatest stress, death of a spouse, and descends to the event that can cause the least, minor violations of the law. With the kind permission of the authors, Thomas Holmes and Richard Rahe of the University of Washington's School of Medicine, I reprint the scale in Appendix M, page 251.

It may well be that a good many of our horrendous traffic fatalities are accident-prone people. Oddly enough, however, some studies have suggested that such individuals are usually very healthy physically. Their personalities have been described as happy-go-lucky, talkative, cheerful, implusive, and somewhat irresponsible. Even odder is the suggestion that they rarely appear to be as tense as the rest of us. It is thought that the emotional key to the accident-prone persons resides in their hostility to and resentment against authority, an emotion developed in rebellion against a rigid and somewhat authoritarian childhood. It is believed that this hostility and resentment can be powerful enough on occasion to cause such individuals to seek escape in irresponsibility, in daring and impulsive behavior that often ends in disaster.

The disease-prone person has not been as clearly delineated as his accident-prone counterpart. The latter may pop in and out of hospitals with astonishing frequency, while the former courts his own disability with poor nutrition, inadequate sleep, and the liberal use of harmful drugs. Both "prones" speed their way to their graves with no deliberate intent and with all outward appearances of wanting to live, of wanting to be healed and healthy. In truth, though, they have given up on life and are hopeless of health and happiness. They have arrived at some strange, internal breaking point.

All in all the whole problem of emotions and disease, mind and body, is fearfully complex. It is not easy to comprehend why, or what caused which, and why some of us maladapt and others stand firm. For example, probably for most of us fear increases the blood flow as we have noted, makes the heart beat faster, and causes a rise in arterial blood pressure to clear the decks for action. But for some people, fear may inhibit the circulatory system, decreasing the blood flow and heart rate, and the individual may faint instead of responding with either fight or flight. This is a sort of psychological "playing possum" in the face of danger. Thus, it cannot be stressed enough that while we may speak in generalities and try to tie labels on this or that emotional disturbance and physical reaction, we must constantly remember that these descriptions do not fit individuals "like a glove." You may have to stretch more than one finger to get the thing on!

While nature makes few judgments and simply allows unsuccessful adaptive behavior to vanish from the face of the earth, we humans enjoy being judge and jury. We tend to deem some behavior or responses as fit and some as not, some as admirable and some as antisocial and even mad upon occasion.

And this thought brings me to a medical problem that tries the patience of us most saintly physicians—the hypochondriac. We even hesitate to say this label out loud! And when we see him coming, we undergo our own variety of emotional stress! However, he is a patient with a patient's basic needs. Often he has not been understood. Physicians worn down by a far-too-intense practice resent his demands when they have little enough time for the seriously ill. He is frequently dismissed with such remarks as "You'll just have to learn to live with it," or "There's really nothing organically wrong with you—it's all in your head," or "You just imagine your symptoms." The hypochondriac's eternal complaint is that no one will listen to him, and his eternal question soon becomes an anxious query, "It isn't all in my head, is it, Doctor?" It is obvious that he has a vital need to be taken seriously, to be reassured. It is obvious that he does really yearn for a way out of very real torment. It is a doctor's responsibility to do his best to meet this need. Not only that, but there is always a trace of unsettling doubt. Have we really, as doctors, done everything to ensure that there is no organic basis for his complaints? To add to our own stress are the many horror tales in the literature of medicine of serious diseases gone undetected in spite of the patient's insistence that something was wrong. Thus a doctor does not pin on the label of hypochondria with an easy mind.

But even with this possibility aside, isn't the hypochondriac really ill? Even when he seems most to be enjoying his aches and pains, isn't he a sick man? Is his a maladaptive response to some emotional need? An unsuccessful coping mechanism? This problem is difficult for doctors to understand sometimes. I once had a colleague say to me in a surprised voice when we discussed such a patient, "He said that he was suffering so much that he'd rather be dead, and he meant it. Yet, there was nothing wrong with him!"

It is far more acceptable in our society to sport physical disabilities than mental ones, and this is what the hypochondriac is desperately trying to do. He is crying out for help in a "respectable" manner, for he knows that he does not feel well although he does not comprehend why or that his feelings are the result of emotional rather than physical imbalances. In any case, his body *is* registering his emotional distress, be it anxiety or guilt or whatever. And unless he is helped to return to a state of hemeostasis, his mode of adaption made more successful, he will spend his precious lifetime suffering one disease symptom after another. He will, if he must, beat his way from one physician's door to another. It is to be hoped that his family or regular doctor can prevent him from having everything jerked out in the course of his rounds!

It should be said that there is danger in simply removing the hypochondriac's crutches without substituting a preferable and healthier means of support. To take away the crutches and command the patient to walk again leaves the poor devil in a precarious position and liable at any moment to lose his balance. If we look upon the hypochondriac's complaints of organic disease as his way of escape from such powerful emotional stresses as feelings of inadequacy, of anxiety, or of guilt, we then can comprehend that to cut off his route of escape is not enough. He must be helped to find a better way. We must tackle the emotional problem itself. Otherwise if we treat, say, his headaches, he may relinquish that symptom only to return with gastrointestinal pains or the like. This unhappy sequence often both angers and unsettles many a busy doctor and makes him doubt his own skills. Thus, the hypochondriac, like Typhoid Mary, carries the bug of emotional distress in and out of doctor's offices across the land!

We should note, too, that hypochondria is not the same as malingering. As with conversion hysteria, the symptoms are very real and very uncomfortable. We should also note that suggestion often plays an important role not only in the development of hypochondria itself but also in the symptoms the patient displays. Frequently there is a family history of this odd and somewhat sad condition, or, at the very least, an intense interest in disease and death in his background. Sometimes hypochondria develops after the patient has suffered an actual, organic illness, especially when convalescence has been prolonged so that he may have found pleasure in unhealthy dependency and the extra attention illness brings. Whatever the case, his treatment usually requires the skills of a psychiatrist. Thus, his problem is really beyond the scope of this book, but I brought him into the discussion for two reasons: one, to indicate that some people do translate the mind's anguish into physical complaints, and, two, because many a truly allergic individual has been dismissed as a hypochondriac, told harshly or gently that his symptoms were all in his head, and sent packing.

And before we move back into our main theme, let us note that oddly enough there is an opposing condition to hypochondria called anosognosia. A person exhibiting this maladaption, unlike the hypochondriac, insists that he is not suffering from an organic disease, that his very real symptoms are minimal. He will insist against all clear evidence to the contrary that his physical problems are all in his mind. I suppose this is a way of shutting out the unpleasant truth, of refusing to admit that one's strength and physical integrity is in any way threatened, not to mention one's life itself. It would seem one more way to escape anxiety.

In summary: the anxious mind can lead us down some strange paths. And we are all vulnerable even though we are not all exposed alike to life and its problems, or to the same environment. Nor do we arrive in this world with the same genetic inheritance. Thus, our responses to stress are as varied as we ourselves and our circumstances are.

This is not to say that emotions and the bodily changes associated with them are abnormal or injurious in themselves. In fact, they are assets to survival. But stress is quantitative as well as qualitative. Prolonged and excessive stress, whether of mind or body, can do harm, can cause actual damage to body systems, can actually alter personality and behavior. Some forms of adaption to stress are uneconomical, unsuccessful. The escape they provide does not enhance and may even threaten the individual's chances for survival.

It is remarkable how our language reflects emotional stresses in physical terms. "He's a pain in the neck," we say. Or, "She rubs me the wrong way." Or, "I always get a lump in my throat at sad movies." Our heads, our hearts, our liver and lungs, our eyes and our skin—just about every organ and body system can mirror in distress the presence of powerful and prolonged emotions, be they fear, anxiety, hostility, guilt, depression, boredom, or loneliness—a host of strong feelings that assail us at sometime or other in our passage from birth to death. Because this is so, holism—the view of the patient as a whole being—makes good sense.

Let us turn now to a fascinating proposition put forth by some proponents of psychosomatic or psychogenic medicine that individuals with certain personality profiles tend to develop certain specific diseases. Then let us consider the mirror image of this concept—that certain diseases can produce certain kinds of personality traits.

3
Does Personality Produce Illness? Or Illness Personality?

Judith P. first came to me with an odd rash covering both her hands. When I took the usual lengthy patient's history, I found there was no record of allergy in her family and that she herself had never as far as she knew suffered any allergy symptoms in the past. I noted that she was a poised and intelligent young woman who appeared perfectly reasonable and, while a little wry about the condition of her hands, not unduly anxious. She spoke lovingly of her children and husband and warmly of their home, the family dog, the pleasantness of their neighborhood, and life in general. Obviously, she harbored no visible stress. Somewhere in our discussion she mentioned that she used both a dishwasher and a clotheswasher, both of which she considered indispensable in a family with three small children. It did not take long to establish that she was using an exceptionally harsh brand of detergent in both machines and that their caustic elements were causing the rash on her hands. My diagnosis was contact dermatitis, due to these chemicals. What emotional overlay I could detect, and it wasn't very great, obviously arose as a result of the mess her hands were in.

"How on earth am I going to cook and clean and change diapers with these!" she exclaimed more than once, holding up her hands.

And that was the extent of her anxiety. So I treated her for contact dermatitis and sent her home quite willing to do without those super-detergents.

Jane T. also came to me with a rash on her hands, but her rash was characterized by intense itching, so much so that she had scratched the back of them raw and scabs had formed in some places. As she talked, I noticed that she dug at her hands constantly. I also noticed that she appeared nervous and tense. As I took her history, her answers to my questions were often mumbled and rambling. She would begin coherently enough, but after the first few words, she appeared to become derailed so to speak, and would go off on tangents.

A woman in her late forties, she had never married, but had chosen instead to stay home to care for her widowed mother. She had a job as a clerk in a shoe store, which she appeared to detest.

"People's feet," she said vaguely. "You know . . . socks."

She brought her mother into the conversation frequently, and several times her voice took on the tones of resentment when she did so.

"She keeps telling me that if I'd just stop scratching my hands, the rash would go away. That's fine, if they aren't your hands and you're not the one itching so awfully! She . . . oh, well, what's the use."

A little later she remarked, "I've often had this rash on my neck and arms before, but never on my hands. It's bad. My job, you know. The customers don't like to see . . . . I told Mother I didn't know what I was going to do. It's not just nonsense! Doctor, I can't stop!" And with that she scratched vigorously.

There was a history of allergy in her family. Her mother had suffered from hay fever for many years and from migraine headaches so fierce that she would withdraw from her family for several days at a time and shut herself in her darkened bedroom.

"When I was a child, I used to think she was trying to get away from me," Jane T. said. "She used to lock the door even. I would cry for her out there in the hall . . . on the floor. Oh, I cried and cried for her to come out and get me. She wouldn't. Not for hours and hours."

So I treated Jane for her eczema, skin-tested her for allergy, and placed her on an elimination diet to see what, if any, foods might be causing her problem. After a few visits, when I felt that we had developed sufficient rapport, I also suggested that she see Dr. S., a psychiatrist in my building. I felt that she needed further insight into her emotional problems and that it was all too likely her allergy could not be controlled until her emotional imbalances were reduced. This is a step I don't take often, for the emotional overlays in allergy are not normally so severe that psychiatric help is necessary.

However, I do not hesitate to recommend that my patients seek such help when it appears that their emotional stress is complex and continuing and that neither self-help nor my shaman-like wisdom seems to diminish their distress. I know that even if I clear up allergy symptoms but emotional difficulties persist, the chances are excellent that the patients will either suffer a relapse of symptoms or come down with a new set or an entirely different illness.

In any case, here we have two patients with similar symptoms but with two totally different causes for them. If I had treated Jane as I treated Judith, (and I'm not talking about medications here), I doubt that I would have solved her allergy problem for very long. Conversely, if I had treated Judith as I had treated Jane, I might have upset her considerably with the suggestion that emotional disturbances were involved in her rash. Thus the psychosomatic approach in medicine requires a bit of caution and good deal of common sense. Like Janus, the problem presents two faces. Some illnesses can in themselves bring on emotional stress, even dramatic changes in personality. By the same token, emotional stress can precipitate some illnesses (perhaps more than we know at present). The recurrent question then, like the old saw of the chicken or the egg, is which comes first? Thus, when you are profoundly depressed, you may feel physically ill. When you are physically ill, you may feel profoundly depressed.

Can we unravel the puzzle of primary cause in order to restore the patient to good health? I think we can, although we may never be wholly certain in the sense of laboratory-certain as to prime cause and precipitating factor. For example, if you know that you will continue in illness if you work under a mean and demanding boss whom you cannot ever sock on the nose to restore a bit of your own, then treatment and good health may depend in part upon a new job under a different kind of boss whose nose does not beg your attention. On the other hand, if your aggressive feelings about your boss are more the result of an extreme irritability caused by an organic illness, say, a liver problem, than of his personality, then it is the disease itself that must be treated to restore emotional balance and health. But, of course, we will not be certain that emotional stress didn't have a hand in the liver problem to begin with. It is not always possible, I believe, to solve this chicken-egg sort of question, so closely are mind and body interwoven.

What is more certain is that continued emotional stress can make restoration of physical health elusive. This, I think, is particularly true in allergy.

This brings us to the working concept of the role of emotional stress in allergy (and other diseases)—the psychosomatic or psychogenic approach. This concept in medicine is as old as the art of healing itself, be it practiced by physician, witchdoctor, or king with his royal touch. The name itself derives from two Greek words—*psyche* 'soul,' and *soma* 'body.' It incorporates the idea that a patient may be ill for reasons other than the presence of a virus or bacterium, or even of an injury incurred. While it has lately been much in vogue, Galen, Greek philosopher and physician of the second century after Christ, estimated that some 60 percent of his patients suffered symptoms born of emotional problems rather than organic disease, an early statistic that some doctors believe compares well with our own modern health problems.

Psychosomatic diseases, and some allergies are strongly suspected of being among them, are considered to be those in which the role of emotional stress is very large, so much so that the disease itself, the organic damage or malfunction, is believed to arise from the physical changes induced by that stress. There is, of course, a good bit of controversy swirling about all this. Some hold the view that most if not all disease other than specifically toxic reactions or specifically genetic disease arises from prolonged emotional stress. Others insist such stress is of minimal significance. I suppose that, as in most situations, the truth resides somewhere in between. In any case, if the reader will allow a little further diversion from the subject of allergy, let's look at some of the diseases often considered psychosomatic plus the proposition put forward by some proponents of this concept that certain kinds of personalities correlate with specific organic illnesses. For example, we've heard much lately about the correlation between a "Type A" personality—considered to be a go-getter, somewhat competitive individual—and heart disease. Many of us are also inclined to associate peptic ulcer with the emotion of anxiety, the worry-worry-worry of our fast-paced modern living.

Doctors have had a unique and now medically famous stomach to study to determine just what kind of physical changes occur during emotional stress. This stomach belonged to Tom, who had the misfortune of swallowing scalding soup as a child. Because his esophagus was destroyed, surgeons cut a large hole in his stomach. This enabled him to taste and chew his food, then spit it directly into his stomach via a tube. Neat, but a bit gaudy! Still, if there is no other way to obtain nourishment, this will do. For Tom, it meant survival and, surprisingly enough, a reasonably normal life. For the doctors, it meant a window into the workings of the stomach. Tom was given a job at the laboratory in exchange for daily observation of his innards.

Among other things, the men of medicine discovered that when Tom felt threatened or afraid, his stomach lost its normal red color as the blood drained away. His stomach became almost white. When he was depressed or felt inadequate and a failure, his stomach action slowed and less acid than normal was released. On the other hand, when he was anxious about something, the mucous membranes of his stomach became swollen and red, his acid secretions markedly greater. If the stress or anxiety had been prolonged, he might well have developed an ulcer. Or if he had inherited the tendency, he might have become sensitized to some food because his stomach was so irritated, and suffered gastrointestinal allergy symptoms. Hostility and anxiety seem to have been the emotions that produced the most potentially harmful alterations in Tom's stomach. There's nothing like a little first-hand knowledge!

Who gets peptic ulcers and the like? It has been suggested that the individual who suffers a good deal from feelings of depression and frustration is the most likely candidate. He is pictured as overly possessive, often jealous, and a bit too fond of accumulating things. He is generally a go-getter, like the cardiac-prone, and while he is aggressive, he seems to have a strong desire to be dependent upon someone. Often he is highly successful in his endeavors, but not necessarily happy in them. In a word, he, too, is a "Type A" and likely to be the harried executive of the TV commercial who is forever bellowing to his secretary to bring the antacid.

Ulcerative colitis, an unpleasant and painful condition characterized by abdominal pain and bloody, mucus-laden diarrhea, is also considered primarily emotional and psychosomatic in origin, although it can also be a response to allergic sensitivity, especially to food. The personality of the colitis victim is believed to be dominated by a strong and continual anger. The sufferer is resentful, depressed and immature, a mother's boy. Suspicious and rigid, he frequently comes from a family situation in which one parent dominates, sometimes brutally so, while the other is submissive, inconsistent, often a martyr. It is suggested that the ulcerative colitis patient is a person who gives up easily, who expresses frustration and hopelessness when events in his life become difficult.

Essential hypertension, which is defined as persistent, above-normal blood pressure for which no organic cause can be found, is believed to be, in good part, a result of emotional stress. It has been suggested that the hypertensive person bottles up strong feelings of hostility, assertiveness, and anxiety, feelings that he apparently cannot openly express or act upon. We all raise our blood pressure on occasion. It is a normal response to stress, but the overly controlled and overly conscientious individual may be just the fellow who should, for the sake of his health, either sock his arrant boss on the nose or go looking for a new job. Preferably both. However, the chances are that he will do all he is asked meekly and resignedly, complain little, swallow his own desire to assert himself, and seethe internally like a volcano. That seething will drive up his blood pressure, and it will persist up there as long as he remains unable to escape from stress. Such an elevated blood pressure may lead to future cardiac problems. Tension and anxiety have such a clear effect on blood pressure that when I find it high for my patients, I retake it after office procedures–skin testing, physical examination, and the like–are completed. It is the only way to be certain that the first reading was not a temporary reflection of these emotions. For example, I have seen a blood pressure of 180/100 drop to 130/80 after the skin tests and shots have ceased on the allergic front!

Allergy, too, especially asthma and eczema, has been considered a psychosomatic disease, as we shall see in later chapters. A good many people, doctors included, harbor a suspicion about the nature of allergy and are even inclined to equate it with hypochondria, as we have noted. There is a somewhat popular notion that much of allergy resides in the heads of its victims. But we shall see.

First, let's go back and flip the coin and take a look at the other face of Janus. This is the other side which proclaims that organic disease in itself can trail emotional stress in its wake, that illness, rather naturally, can cause emotional stress.

We have discussed how emotions can alter the biochemistry of the body, so it should not be difficult to comprehend that the biochemistry of the body can influence the working of the mind. Emotions are organic phenomena. They arise from bodily changes. Obviously then, physical stress can cause emotional stress. When we discussed the conversion hysteria of the young paratroopers of World War II, we noted that they suffered extreme exhaustion coupled with malnutrition as well as constant and profound anxiety. Malnutrition, vitamin deficiency, and inadequate sleep are excellent examples of bodily conditions that can influence the mind, and much laboratory research has been done to illustrate this. For example, striking psychic disturbances can result from hunger, ranging from hallucinations verging on veritable "trips" to total passivity and depression. Pellagra, for instance, a disease usually associated with protein deficiency, can produce a psychosis characterized by depression, anxiety, weakness, a short attention span, and confusion. Malnutrition during early childhood may modify the growth and maturation of the brain, resulting in retardation and personality disturbances. Vitamins play a vital role in the biochemistry of the nervous system and their deficiency can lead to emotional and personality disturbances. As a matter of interest, most of us know that iodine deficiency can lead to goiter, but probably few of us realize that it can also cause mental retardation in children. It is also believed that there may be some connection between this condition and schizophrenia.

To add to the litany of the mental and emotional effects of bodily ills, some interesting work has been done lately on the relationship of relative hypoglycemia (drop in blood sugar level) and emotional disturbances. The condition has no organic cause yet discovered other than a too-high carbohydrate food intake and/or too much caffeine. Along with such somatic symptoms as weakness, headache, rapid heart beat, chronic indigestion, backache, and joint pains, the sufferer often exhibits such emotional distress as anxiety, irritability, depression, confusion, phobias, crying jags, and even antisocial and suicidal tendencies.

Sleep disturbances can be both a symptom of and a cause for emotional stress. We know that sleep deprivation not only brings about bodily changes but also affects observable behavior. One experiment records that a group of military officers were given staff work tasks alternated with shooting on a rifle range. While this went on for several days, they were allowed no sleep or relaxation, no coffee or other stimulants, no smoking or walking about to keep themselves awake. Not only did actual biochemical somatic changes take place, but they also suffered considerable emotional disturbances—as can be imagined!

Depression and fatigue are often indications of illness, sometimes of such serious organic problems as cancer, anemia, or congestive heart failure. Frequently, even during mild illnesses, patients become depressed out of all proportion to the severity of their health problem. Some patients even become angry and resentful, hating to find themselves physically vulnerable. And fear, especially, is a wholly normal response to many physical ailments. Most of us are afraid of pain, and I would suppose that most of us, too, are afraid of death. When sickness strikes, it is not surprising that we should feel anxious, frightened, and depressed as we anticipate, perhaps, these contingencies.

Disease states are not the only factors to generate emotional stress. I have long been interested in the role some common pollutants of our modern environment play in mental ill health. By directly affecting the biochemistry of our bodies, such pollutants also affect our minds and are reflected in our behavior and personality. Lead and mercury, for instance, two extremely toxic heavy metals, can not only cripple us physically but they can alter who we are. The damage they may do to both body and mind can range from the subtle and temporary to the massive and permanent. Early symptoms of an abnormal body burden of lead, for instance, may be extreme irritability, restlessness, compulsiveness, an inability to concentrate. Some of us are more susceptible than others to such toxic substances, and thus may be affected by amounts in the environment that do not cause symptoms in the general population. A study made of two Swiss prisons found that a good many inmates not only had high body burdens of lead, but they also had more difficulty than normal persons excreting it. Thus, they accumulated more lead than normal, although they may have suffered the same exposure. The study suggested that there may be some relationship between this susceptibility and the antisocial behavior that led them to the prison gates. Since the lead body burden of inner city children tends to be higher than for youngsters in general, we can speculate that there may be some correlation between such lead burdens and the higher crime and juvenile delinquency rates of our cities.

Interesting, too, is the suggestion of a West Coast chemist that there may be a relationship between the higher rate of suicides in his area than the rate in the East and the greater hydrogen sulfide pollution from the region's pulp paper mills. Depression, the emotional state that brings far too many people to the point of desiring death, is probably a major disease. There is increasing evidence that it may result from a decreased production of catecholamines (the chemicals that transmit messages to the brain and play an essential role in emotional stress). Some researchers and physicians believe that there is a hereditary factor in the physical production of these chemicals, and that, oddly enough, this production follows a biological rhythm. The sufferer from such decreased production may feel most depressed in the morning and least toward evening. Also, this psychosis strikes commonly when a person is in the mid-thirties, perhaps when such production is on the wane for one reason or another. The West Coast chemist's question is this: can hydrogen sulfide trigger or incude such lowered production of the catecholamines, especially among the genetically vulnerable? Thus, again, we can speculate about whether there are pollutants in our environment to account, at least in part, for some of our mental illnesses.

By now, I perceive that you are shuffling your feet and tapping your fingers. Come, come, Doc, what has all this to do with allergy?

Well, let me pose a proposition, one that I can't answer at the moment, but find interesting to consider. Both allergy diseases and aberrant behavior and emotional stresses appear to be increasing in our modern, technological society. So are pollution and the use of thousands of new chemicals, many of them man-made and not found in nature. Is it possible that we are producing stimuli, chemical and psychosocial, which can produce in turn body alterations that affect both the nervous system and allergic sensitivity?

But you are right, that is the subject of another book. However, before we move on to connect allergy to emotions and vice versa, let us take a brief look at the role of our "biological clocks" in both, and in our lives as well. It is fascinating that we do all march to our own drummer in illness as in health, in distress as in joy.

4
Biological Clocks in Illness and in Health

We are more closely bound to our world and the universe than many of us know, for all living things follow rhythmic cycles as though programmed by some mysterious force. Powerful waxing and waning of body and brain biochemistry follows ancient biological rhythms, for we are attuned to the turning of the earth, the alterations of day and night, the monthly phases of the moon, the yearly seasons. "Biological clocks" set deep in our marrow, governed by endogenous factors whose origin and nature we do not yet thoroughly understand, direct the physical and emotional changes we must make on our journey from birth to death. We do come into the world to the beat of our own drummer, and we march in step until the day we die.

The most pronounced of our "biological clocks" is the rhythm of our daily lives, the circadian cycle of approximately 24 hours associated with day and night. We rise to it in the morning as the solar day begins, and we go to rest to its beat in the evening as darkness comes. We are not the same, however, from hour to hour, even though the pattern of the inner rhythm we follow is generally akin to the pattern of the rhythm of the day before. For instance, we know that our body temperature fluctuates by almost several degrees, peaking in afternoon or evening for the day-hunter or individual who is active during the daylight and sleeps at night. Night-hunters, on the other hand, may peak later in the evening. In one study, it was discovered that people who slept well at night usually had a body temperature that approached or was "normal" by the time they habitually rose in the morning, whereas the individual who was a poor sleeper had a body temperature still below "normal" at rising time, and, as a matter of fact, it was still working its way up to "normal" for several hours after the person was up and doing. This may well account for those early morning grumps and fatigue. Unhappily for many of us, while we are changing, our workaday world remains rigid. We are expected to all operate the same, when in actuality we cannot. And should not!

Body temperature is not the only changing physical function during our circadian cycle. Hormone production, the ability to synthesize food, production of excretory constituents—a host of physiological processes change from hour to hour to follow our body's particular rhythm. And even as physical alterations occur, so do mental ones. We may be able to learn more easily during certain hours of the day, and we may be somewhat stupid and disorganized at others. We may be eager, alert, and confident in the morning and depressed and negative by late afternoon.

Strangely enough, even if we were isolated in a windowless room where light and darkness played no role and no mechanical watch or clock informed us of the hour, we would still follow our own individual rhythm, although it might deviate a little from the solar 24 hour day or the lunar (24.8) cycle. Like those astonishing time-lapse photographs that follow a plant through its daily gyrations—leaves rising and opening expectantly, then drooping and closing at the coming of darkness—our pulse rate, blood pressure, body temperature, blood sugar levels, breathing, and the like are altered to the rhythm of our "clock" or "clocks." And our ability to function physically and mentally depends on these alterations within us. During some periods of our cycle, our bodies and minds are at their peak, at others at their nadir. It is well to pay heed to our "clock," for there are times in the day when we are all but invincible, and there are times in the day when we are very vulnerable.

For example, experiments with rats have shown that during the period when their "biological clock" is calling for rest, a loud noise doesn't much disturb them; but the same intensity of noise during a period of activity can send them into convulsions and may even be fatal. The tolerance or vulnerability of the rats to noise is apparently related to the rhythm of their adrenal gland cycle.

We can even take advantage of this alteration in vulnerability in our war against the insect world. We have discovered, for example, that exposure to an insecticide at dawn will kill only about

10 percent of a given beetle population, whereas the same exposure a few hours later will kill some 90 percent of them. It is easy to see that testing of a commercial insecticide could yield erroneous predictions of the product's effectiveness! And in fact, a large margin of error can occur when drugs are tested for efficacy and/or safety if the biological rhythms of laboratory animals are ignored.

Translated into human terms, the alterations of vulnerability during the circadian cycle can be extremely important in drug treatment and the scheduling of surgery. At certain hours of the day we may be more resistant to a drug than at others; therefore it may be less effective. By the same token, at certain hours of the day we may be much more vulnerable to toxic qualities of a drug, even dangerously so. As for surgery, it is traditionally scheduled in the early morning, yet this may be the most vulnerable time for some people, a time when their reaction to stress could be quite low. Lately, with our increasing awareness of the vital role of "biological clocks," some medical men are suggesting that surgery be performed according to a profile of the individual patient's circadian rhythm. This would ensure that the patient would undergo the stress of an operation at that point in his circadian rhythm when his body could best handle it. We do know that we are most likely to depart this world in the early morning hours between three and four o'clock. Oddly enough, as every obstetrician knows to his occasional dismay, we are also most likely to be born during these inconvenient hours.

Can our circadian rhythm be changed? Can our "biological clock" be reset as measured by the solar day or mechanical clocks?

Definitive answers applicable to everyone probably do not yet exist, but isolation studies have produced some interesting results. Deprived of the cycle of light and darkness and in the absence of a watch or clock, individuals tend to lengthen their circadian rhythm of activity and rest periods above the 24-hour solar day. Initially, there may be a period in which rhythms oscillate, but after this span of instability, the circadian rhythm stabilizes again in what is called a "free-running" rhythm. For instance, individuals who took up residence in caves for extended periods of time and without exterior cues for activity and rest, found themselves going to bed later each day and rising correspondingly later on the next day. One man who spent 127 days in a cave began his stay by being all out of phase. He was active, for instance, for 10 hours, then slept 9, for a 19-hour day, and then was active for 18 hours and slept 35 for a 53-hour cycle. However, during the last half of his stay underground, he settled into a 25.2-hour circadian rhythm.

Jet lag has long been of interest to researchers. Persons who fly east-west from one time zone to another exhibit a slowing of response and mental alertness, an inability to concentrate, and feelings of fatigue. No jet lag occurs on north-south flights of equal length within the same time zone. Thus, there is some physical and mental hazard to flying in the jet age, for the air traveler (and pilot and crew) can get out of synchronization with his new environment or external time. Thus, his circadian rhythm may call for sleep at noon in Rome or Tokyo, even as his business or social obligations call for alertness. It may take him as long as a week to readjust his rhythm to the new "time." There are some rather serious implications for our diplomats–State Department officials on their various "shuttles," for instance–in the physical and psychological effects of jet lag.

Shift workers face much the same problem in readjustment of their circadian rhythms and external clock time. In one survey, such workers were found to have a higher-than-normal incidence of ulcers; and in a recent study of a thousand workers in Rhone valley industries, it was found that some 45 percent could not adjust to a weekly rotation of shift, while some 34 percent were incapable of adjusting to a two-day rotation. The circadian body temperature rhythms failed to adapt to such work-time alterations. Even in those shift workers who apparently can adapt to changing work regimens, long-term health problems may ensue, both mental and physical. One doctor has suggested that jet pilots on east-west runs show signs of premature aging, for instance, and laboratory studies on animals of such phase shifts indicate that periods of resistance and/or vulnerability to toxic substances change drastically. Such phase shifts are a type of stress, with all that this may mean for our emotional and physical health.

But there is a transposition here perhaps, for it may be that emotional stress can alter circadian rhythm. At least in animal experiments emotional stress has been reported to alter body-temperature circadian rhythm. In one experiment with monkeys, for example, the subjects with implanted sensors to measure body and brain functions were taught to push a lever to avoid noxious stimuli. They soon learned to keep one paw on this lever. Experimenters then fixed the lever in such a way that while the monkeys could see it, they could not touch it. Even though no noxious stimuli were employed, the poor monkeys became frantic. Within two weeks, their brain-temperature cycle altered as much as half an hour a day. Some developed 48-hour brain temperature rhythms. Physical symptoms of their emotional stress included sores, wheezing, bloody stools, and skin ulcers. Mental symptoms included psychotic behavior.

Circadian rhythm is not the only internal timepiece that we possess. We also follow monthly, seasonal, and annual cycles. Women, for instance, are very much aware of their monthly cycle, which affects not only their bodies but their emotions as well. Husbands commonly are also aware of the female monthly rhythm, sometimes to their dismay. Women aren't alone in this, however. Men also follow a less conspicuous but none the less definite monthly cycle. As far back as the seventeenth century a doctor, Sanctorious, discovered that men alter their body weight by as much as one or two pounds during a four-week period. A scientist in Antarctica for a year of research discovered that his bedtime pattern would alter every 28 days. For 28 days he would go to bed a little later each evening, then revert at the end of this period to his original bedtime and start the cycle all over again.

We also possess seasonal and annual cycles, although not as much is known about these rhythms. Most of us, however, have experienced and been aware of the bounding joy and energy of springtime and the depressed mood of late fall. It is interesting to note that our thyroid glands actually produce a "summer hormone" that helps reduce our body heat. And, statistically, we know that in the temperate zone suicides are highest in May, arteriosclerosis deaths in January, and accidental deaths in July and August. Researchers are quick to point out, of course, that certain cultural customs—automobile trips, swimming, and boating, for example—occur in the main in July and August, which could account for the last statistic to a large extent.

One fascinating seasonal "winter madness" occurs among Eskimos in the Arctic Zone. This odd psychosis, which can last for hours or days, has been called "arctic hysteria." Dr. Joseph Bohlen of the

Univeristy of Wisconsin studied ten Eskimos at Wainwright, Alaska. For periods of ten days during each of the four seasons, he took urine samples and recorded blood pressure, oral temperature, and pulse every two hours. He also had his subjects take hand-grip and eye-coordination tests. His most interesting finding was that every one of his subjects exhibited an annual rhythm in calcium excretion, excreting eight to ten times more calcium during the winter than in summer. Since calcium is important to the proper functioning of the nervous system, especially in the transmission of nerve messages, it is possible to theorize that here may be the basis for "arctic hysteria." We do know that calcium deficiency can cause hyperirritability.

Since the nervous system is affected by physiological fluctuations, we may be more vulnerable to emotional stress at certain times during our biological cycles than at others. As long ago as 1929, Dr. Rex B. Hersey made a study of workers in an industrial plant. He followed them about their daily tasks for many weeks, asking a list of questions. He discovered that over a four-to-six-week cycle, these men exhibited a somewhat regular pattern of emotional alterations. They moved almost imperceptibly from an easy-going, calm mood to a period of irritability and tension. So gradual were these changes in mood that the workers themselves were not aware of their altering emotional casts. If we had patience and objectivity enough, it is probable that we could record enough data about our own biological rhythms to be able to recognize our emotional fluctuations.

Where we stand in life, our physical age, has a good bit to do with these fluctuations also. For example, depression, anxiety, irritibility are often linked to "change of life" of the middle years. Physical symptoms are also connected to this time of decreasing hormone production–headaches, joint pains, muscle tenderness. Because some menopausal symptoms are occasionally mistaken for allergy and/or because allergy symptoms often seem to be aggravated by the hormonal and emotional disorders of this period, I treat a good many women who are struggling through the menopause. It is odd, but I've found that it is frequently difficult to obtain a coherent history of their complaints and health backgrounds. They seem unable to concentrate on their chief symptoms but rather tend to wander from one vague complaint to another as though totally overwhelmed by unhappiness and anxiety. Often enough, their problems, or at least some of them, are due to allergy, but this fact tends to get lost in the prolixity of their sorrows.

On the other hand, pregnancy, a time of massive hormonal production, may be emotionally the least stressful period in a woman's life. We often remark how beautiful and serene a pregnant woman appears. This is the case because both physically and emotionally she is at a peak. However, sadly enough, she often must pay for her bliss with postpartum "blues," the great crying jag and depression that frequently follows on the heels of giving birth and marks a return to normal hormonal production. Thus, emotionally, women rise and fall like Rome through the fulfillment of this vital role. (Unhappily, I must add that often pregnancy ushers in the beginning of allergy symptoms!)

Before we leave the role of our "biological clocks" on our emotional life, let us note the extraordinary story of Mary Lamb, sister of the famous English essayist Charles Lamb. Perhaps, in truth, I should acknowledge that the story is really his, for he is the selfless hero. This case illustrates clearly how recurrent emotional disturbances, including mild mental illnesses, often exhibit periodic or rhythmic fluctuations.

Mary Lamb's case is one of the more famous accounts in the literature of periodic psychosis. In one of her cyclical attacks of insanity she stabbed her own mother to death. It was said that she was "worn down to a state of extreme misery by attention to needle work by day and to her mother by night," for the mother was an invalid and evidently needed much care. Charles Lamb, who had himself once become so mentally disturbed as to have been confined for a short time, managed to have his sister placed in his custody. For the rest of his life he had to deal with her recurring bouts of psychosis, some 38 all told, which increased with age with shorter intervals of normality between attacks. At the early signs of an approaching seizure, he would place her in a straitjacket, and she would be rushed to the hospital. In between attacks she was entirely normal, a highly intelligent woman with many friends. A writer herself, she produced a number of stories, some in conjunction with her more famous brother. In the end, she outlived him by some 13 years, dying at the reasonably ripe age of 83. In the 50 years that she suffered from cyclical psychosis, she apparently suffered no physical or mental deterioration. It may be simply that somehow, for some reason, a biological clock had gone awry.

Biological rhythms then play a role in emotional stress, which in turn may affect the allergic individual's tolerance to allergenic substances in the environment. But our biological clocks may play an even more direct role than this in allergy illnesses, for allergy symptoms, particularly those of the asthmatic individual, appear to follow circadian rhythm. Asthma often strikes its victims at night at a time when adrenal corticoid levels are at their lowest. There apparently is also a histamine release cycle, for hay fever victims and individuals allergic to house dust frequently suffer their most severe symptoms in the evening just before bedtime. In a study of patients allergic to penicillin it was discovered that their reactions to the antibiotic were greatest at around eleven in the evening, a time when corticoid production was lowest. Thus, allergic persons may be far more vulnerable to allergens in the environment at certain times of the day and, perhaps, of the month or year.

The fact that our bodies follow such rhythms of strength and vulnerability is of great importance in the treatment of disease, as we have seen. For instance, adrenal hormones are the substances most effective in the treatment of severe asthma; thus, when the body's own production of these hormones is low, medication supplements to prevent asthma attacks or to mitigate their severity are given. In the light of our present knowledge of the circadian rhythm of adrenal function it then makes sense that there are optimum times to administer these powerful steroid drugs. These drugs do not actually cure asthma; they control it. And they present health problems in their own right; thus it is vital to employ them when it is absolutely necessary, when they will do the most good, in as small a quantity as possible. For example, instead of the daily doses of steroid drugs once given youngsters suffering from severe asthma, careful observation of the adrenal cycle has resulted in what is called alternate-day therapy. This procedure reduces the risk of side effects such as stunted growth and delayed maturation in children and the appearance of the typical "moon face" of steroid treatment.

It is noteworthy that patients on corticosteroid drugs may need to have their dosage increased when they are stressed by additional illness, surgery, or even emotional upset. Why? Because their own adrenal function may be decreased by long-term employment of these drugs so that their bodies cannot handle additional stress on their own. This is one reason why the prescription of such powerful drugs must be weighed with great care and benefits set against possible harmful effects.

The importance of adrenal hormones on physical and mental health within the circadian cycle has been well established in many animal studies, but we have not found the "clock" responsible for this vital function. For some time it was thought that if the adrenal glands were removed, the circadian rhythm of cell division would cease. However, this appears not to be the case, although such division does slow markedly in such tissues as the skin. Not only that, but adrenal glands isolated in solution still pour forth their hormones in an unmistakable rhythm, which makes the existence of a "master clock" a puzzle. Yet, to further confuse the problem, patients who suffer brain damage or malfunction such as confusion or coma exhibit altered circadian rhythm of the adrenal glands, a finding that has led the searchers for a "master clock" to the hypothalamus and its relationship to the pituitary gland, the mighty peanut of our brains.

Obviously we still have a lot to learn about biological clocks. We do know with certainty that they are vital to our well-being, both physical and emotional.

5
The Effects of Weather on Allergy and Emotions

While we physically and mentally follow the beat of our unheard biological rhythms, the world outside impinges upon us powerfully. We must adapt to its external vagaries even as we strive to retain homeostasis to our own internal tune. Weather is not only one of the most fickle of the factors that require us constantly to adapt, but it also plays a very large role in our ability to function, a much larger role than many of us realize.

Weather has always intruded into the affairs of mankind. Every schoolchild learns that "Old Man Winter," Russian-style, foiled Napoleon's vaulting ambition. Even though the courage of the people and soldiers at Stalingrad did much to turn the tide against Hitler's equally mad lust for power, again the Russian winter played a vital role. Weather, it would seem, has played an equally capricious part in man's capricious warring.

In our more mundane affairs weather affects our ability to react both physically and mentally to external influences. Perhaps we recognize this subconsciously, for we obviously accord weather a large place in our daily concerns. If we do nothing else, we discuss it endlessly. In truth, what happens to our environment, as we are just now beginning to realize, very much affects the affairs of humankind. Even minute changes in the atmosphere, for instance, may change our lives, at least temporarily. For example, when a volcano, Tambora, erupted some one hundred years ago, it affected not only English weather a hemisphere away, but also disrupted the nation's economic and social fabric and, no doubt, strained English health and emotional well-being. How? The pollutants spewed forth from the eruption affected weather worldwide, causing poor crops in England. In turn, the price of flour rose precipitously, with all that such an increase could mean for the country's inhabitants—malnutrition for the poor, emotional stress for other large segments of the population, and the like.

When Kenneth E. F. Watt of the University of California cites this example in his book *Principles of Environmental Science,** he warns that this sort of volcano-spawned chain of events can be considered a prototype of a pattern our increasing pollution of the atmosphere can bring about—may, in fact, already be bringing about. If we subtly alter the weather, we may not only alter our ability to raise food, but we may also be altering our very selves, for our physical, emotional, and social aspects are tenaciously cohesive. For instance, the automobile is a way of life in our nation. It actually underpins our society. Without cars, we could not live as we do. To make engines run a bit smoother, we put lead in gasoline. This lead is spewed out, in part, in automobile exhausts, and where traffic is heavy, it accumulates in the air and soil. Since traffic is heavy in urban areas, inner-city people are most heavily exposed to this pollutant. Lead affects health in various ways, one of which, as was mentioned earlier, is damage to the nervous system, causing aberrant, sometimes violent behavior. We can speculate that perhaps some of urban crime may be a direct result of lead pollutions in the environment. But again, this is a subject for another book. Let us define what aspects of the weather most affect allergy and emotions.

Temperature, humidity, barometric pressure, and wind appear to play the greatest role in our physical and mental well-being. However, it has been suggested recently that electromagnetic waves and positive and negative ions may also have some effect upon us, especially upon our emotions. Certainly allergy is affected by temperature changes and humidity. Alterations in weather place a strain upon us physically as we seek to adapt to new external conditions. Unless they are extraordinarily intense, it is not so much the conditions themselves that stress us—whether cold or heat, low humidity or high, and so on—as it is the fluctuations in these factors requiring physiological changes on our part. Once our bodies have adapted to new weather conditions, unless, of course, they are extreme, the element of stress recedes. For this

*New York: McGraw-Hill, 1973.

reason, fluctuations in weather conditions often act as triggers to set off symptoms in the allergic individual, especially symptoms of asthma and rhinitis.

Weather also affects the allergic person directly. The individual sensitive to mold, for example, is not going to do very well during warm, damp weather during which mold populations are likely to explode. Low humidity and hot, dry weather, on the other hand, can often make asthma worse since such weather tends to dry mucous plugs in the bronchi, making it more difficult to expel stale air. Cold, long winters increase the allergic person's exposure to house dust and furnace fumes, but, conversely, an early frost puts an end to pollination. Thus, it really becomes a matter of take it or leave it for the allergic individual. His problems will depend in part upon what allergens he is sensitive to and what the weather's effect on those allergens will be. However, there is one factor that is somewhat universal here—areas of storm tracks with their rapidly changeable weather patterns are the least healthy areas for allergic persons, especially those who suffer from respiratory symptoms.

For example, we know that in such areas the abrupt and often violent changes of barometric pressure and temperature can trigger asthma attacks. We do not thoroughly understand the mechanism involved, although we do know that some people are hypersensitive to cold and heat. Since faulty adrenal function frequently plays a vital role in the production of asthma, there may be an inability on the part of the asthmatic individual to adjust to sudden weather changes. Whether such an inability to adjust internal temperature and other physiological functions to meet changing external conditions arises in the nervous system or because of hormonal imbalance is not known with any certainty.

Man has observed, however, that weather changes very clearly affect his behavior and feelings. One aspect, the föhn—or foehn, as it is sometimes spelled—wind has long intrigued layman and scientist alike. The föhn is a hot, dry wind or dry air storm that occurs when a strong wind blows over mountains and is dragged downward on the lee side. Indians call it a "chinook" or snow-eater in the Rocky Mountain area. In California it is the Santa Ana wind, in France, the mistral, in Israel the sharav, in Switzerland, the föhn. By whatever name, it does affect human emotions, perhaps because positive ions build up in the atmosphere just before the winds arrive. People become tense, irritable, depressed, so much so that a Swiss study indicated that during the föhn wind, suicide rates and admissions to mental hospitals rise markedly. In Israel, statistics demonstrate that when this wind blows, some young people exhibit violent behavior, while their elders become tense and depressed. It has been said that during the period just before the dry air storm, people frequently exhibit abnormal behavior and there is a noticeable increase in crime and violence.

Possible effects of the ionization quality, if it can be called that, of the atmosphere have been the subject of much speculation and some research. Results to date have been inconclusive. Some scientists believe that atmospheric ions have a good deal to do with human behavior, while others theorize that electromagnetic fields play a role. Such ions are charged atmospheric particles, atoms or molecules, which are unstable because they possess either more or fewer electrons than normal. Those with an electronic excess are negative ions and those with a deficit are positive. Ions are formed in the atmosphere when oxygen atoms are struck by cosmic rays, by light particles, or by other molecules. In the soil, they are formed by radioactive bombardment. Actually, ions apparently benefit living things. Studies of mice kept in an atmosphere containing no ions demonstrated that the mice were twice as susceptible to flu virus as were control mice. Plants set in such a "dead" atmosphere show growth retardation. Ions are destroyed quickly in the atmosphere when they collide with other particles or the earth itself. Pollutant particles, for instance, deionize; thus in a room filled with tobacco smoke (particles) the air soon becomes "dead" with all that this may mean for persons therein. The "smoke-filled rooms" of politics may not offer the optimum environment to conduct the business of the people. That environment may, in fact, tend to stupefy, a fact which may explain a good deal of what goes wrong with the conduct of some of our affairs.

Ions have been associated with mood changes as well as with growth and susceptibility. In an atmosphere with a superfluity of positive ions, the serotonin (a hormone that affects the nervous system) level rises. Serotonin has also been associated with physical alterations, such as retardation of healing and constriction of blood vessels It also alters mood, causing irritability, aggression, an increased sensitivity to pain. Thus, when the föhn wind blows—increasing quantities of positive ions in the atmosphere, which, in turn, raise the level of serotonin in human bloodstreams—it may hold an explanation for the aberrant behavior that apparently correlates with this weather phenomenon.

Negative ions, on the other hand, have been associated with a sense of well-being and a tranquilizing effect. However, although interesting to contemplate, none of these suggested possibilities have yet been conclusively "proved." All we know is that the weather plays a role in our emotional life as well as our physical health.

The "long hot summers" of our inner cities, for example, have added both physical and mental stress to already badly stressed urban dwellers. Urban police forces stand by when temperatures rise, for heat stress causes predictable outbreaks of violence as well as physical alterations such as increased heartbeat and respiration. Laboratory studies with rats have also demonstrated that as temperature rises, learning ability decreases. Heat stress alters body chemistry; for example, it promotes an increased production of aldosterone, a substance secreted by the adrenal cortex that controls the metabolism of sodium chloride and potassium and the release of growth hormone that produces retention of salt and water. It is worth noting that often heat stroke victims exhibit psychotic behavior as an early symptom of their physical damage.

Now that we have touched upon some general influences upon both allergy and emotional stress, let us turn to the allergic patient himself. Who is he? What bothers him? How does he mirror his problems? How does he feel about himself?

6

Personality Types in My Office

I suppose that every emotion possible to the human species has been exhibited at some time or other by my various patients, but those that confront me most frequently are anxiety and depression—a situation which is not surprising, considering that many of my patients have been suffering chronic, annoying (at the very least) symptoms for some time. Small wonder that they feel anxious and unhappy. And this is especially true for the allergic patient whose well-meaning (?) friends have intimated that most of his problem may be in his imagination, that all he needs to do is buck up and stop worrying so much about himself. To add to his distress, his own doctor may have come to the conclusion that nothing is organically wrong with him and may have even hinted that he is suffering from "nerves." This situation can be devastating. Often such patients arrive in my office on the defensive, ready to defend themselves against a verdict that nothing is wrong with them really, that their symptoms are "all in their heads." A patient with such a background may also get quite angry when skin tests do show that he has an allergy. "Why didn't the doctors find it earlier?" he will demand. "Why did they keep giving me such a runaround?"

Since I deal to a great extent with allergic children (my training in allergy followed my pediatric training), I see all sorts of emotional stresses among my young patients—and incipient personality disorders as well. Fear and anxiety are rather naturally foremost among the emotions they exhibit. It is natural to be afraid of the doctor, his office, and the staff of strangers, of medicine and especially of shots, of all the glittering, strange paraphernalia of the treatment room. I admit to a few pangs of unease myself when a health problem takes me to one of my colleagues. Being allergic myself, I take a number of shots. Knowing my marked antipathy to this procedure, my staff leave syringes on my desk and draw straws to see who gets to "stick" me. On occasion they bring in a tearful young patient to gloat over the doctor getting back some of his own medicine. On such occasions I roar even louder than usual. How sadistic children are! And nurses!

Of course, I do my best to dispel this normal stress among my young patients. No doctor wants youngsters to begin screaming at the mere sight of him. I often employ a little verse:

There's nothing to fear,
Dr. Frazier is here!

And always I discuss the procedure we will go through and why. Even the very small child can become interested in the process of finding out what is causing him to sneeze or wheeze, have stomachaches or itching. Normally, the mildly apprehensive child doesn't cringe when I examine him, and when it's all over, he isn't angry with me. Often enough, he will proudly state that it didn't hurt much. Often enough he'll give me a hug before he leaves. Our rapport is established. All is well. Actually, it continues to amaze me how quickly youngsters return to normal, shed their fear and apprehension, and laugh again at my jokes. When the nurse offers a toy, of course the process is speeded a bit.

It is the child who relentlessly clings to his mother, especially if he is over five years old, who appears so panic-stricken that he cannot be diverted, or who is so overactive and restless that he cannot sit still, or who bites his fingers and hands constantly, or who is obviously timid and tense—he is a child that I immediately suspect of having real emotional problems of one kind or another. Anger, too, can sometimes indicate unhealthy emotional pressures. Frequently, the mother is the target of a youngster's rage. The child who hits out at her, who strikes at her face with his fist or who has a temper tantrum in my office, especially if he is over four, is indicating some deep-seated tension. If the mother simply remarks, "That's not nice," I can be sure this child is on his way to personality disturbance. While breath-holding during a temper tantrum or bout of crying (and there are days when my office rings with shrieks and sobs) is a frequent manifestation among my youngest patients, in older children it may signal extreme frustration. Or it may simply be an attention-getting device. At the other extreme is the child who sits very quietly while his mother does all the talking; he, too, may be displaying some emotional problem. For instance, I have noticed that frequently the overprotected boy is usually very passive and apt to be obese.

One way to discover what is bothering a child is to give it dolls or puppets to play with. By labeling the dolls "Mommy" doll, "Daddy" doll, "Brother Jim" doll, and the like, the child may act out some of the conflicts in the family and his own inner feelings. I vividly recall a child I'll call Mary whom I treated during my pediatric residency. Calling one of the dolls Mary, her own name, she put Mary to bed; but poor Mary couldn't sleep because "Uncle Jim," "Uncle Bob," "Uncle Tom," a string of "Uncles" came calling on Mommy doll. Alas, the child's mother wasn't married at the moment. That parade of gentlemen friends must have been emotionally traumatic for this little girl.

If one has the time and patience to sit quietly and watch children act out stories with the dolls or puppets, one can learn a great deal about a child's emotional conflicts and relationships within the family. If, for instance, Mommy doll takes a beating, there is probably something radically wrong in the child's life. The child's use of such words as "bad," "good," "witch," "angel," and the like as he plays with the dolls also provides clues to his feelings.

Another excellent way to elicit free expression from children is to provide them with quantities of drawing paper and crayons, then encourage a running commentary about the pictures they make. Who is that? Mommy? What's she doing? And so on.

None of this is one hundred percent certain, especially when a child is not emotionally upset, for the well-loved child usually has nothing very urgent to express and simply plays happily. Still if we are alert, we may find clues to very real problems. And if their emotional stress is having an effect on allergy symptoms, such clues may be invaluable.

When it comes to personality types, while I have found that few of my allergy patients, young or old, fall neatly into cut-and-dried categories, certain recognizable characteristics often do appear. Trying to pinpoint personality can be somewhat difficult in any case. There are a number of descriptions assigning this and that characteristic to this or that type of personality. Some divide people into two slots such as Type A and Type B personalities, while others use more pigeon holes for people. Dr. Gerald D. Bell, Professor of Organizational Behavior in the School of Business at the University of North Carolina, delineates six different pure personality types in his book *The Achievers.* With his kind permission I would like to borrow them and take them into my office to see if I can try them on my patients for a proper fit. Let us remember, though, that few of us fit the pure type. Most of us possess attributes of several or all, although frequently one set of traits dominates all the rest so that we can say, aha, he is a type so-and-so personality.

The Commander

Dr. Bell says of him:

> The commander needs to control whatever situation he confronts, dominate every group he is in, and live an orderly, systematic life. He dislikes ambiguity and uncertainty. He sees his world in clear-cut categories, and approaches new situations in a dogmatic and stubborn manner.

In my office he is brisk. "You see, Doc, here is the way it is. When I eat tomatoes, I wheeze. Now I know I shouldn't eat them, but you know how it is . . . ."

If he misses several weeks between his desensitization shots, shots which are gradually increased in strength to raise the allergic person's tolerance to such allergens as pollen, he will demand, nay, command, the nurse who gives the shots not to drop back on the dosage just because he's "missed a few." The flustered nurse runs to me: "What shall I do?" Now I know he's going to be hard to reason with, so if I'm sure it isn't going to harm him, I tell her loudly, hoping he can hear, "Go ahead. If he passes out, get him out of the office quick!" However, if I believe he has to drop back on the dosage, I stand firm and he will eventually give in. But not without a struggle!

He is the fellow who, even if he has been handed a typewritten list of the foods he is to avoid to control his allergy, will draw his chair up to my desk, clear away some of my things to make room, pull pen and pad from his pocket and briskly set about jotting down all his forbidden foods. "Let's see now, Doc, no eggs, huh?"

Frequently the commander is widely read and does not hesitate to keep you abreast of all the latest medical discoveries and proper treatments for his particular ailment. I usually reply, "Oh, yes, that was new several years ago. The post mortem examinations of those who succumbed were quite interesting." If he persists, "Aw come on, Doc, you're kidding. It's supposed to be a breakthrough," I reply, "I know the article you're talking about. It was written by a friend of mine (and it usually was), but it's still experimental. I wouldn't use it on myself and I won't use it on any of my patients!" The commander has to be shown, firmly shown, that you know your business. If he takes the treatment out of your hands, you're a goner.

He is one of the most difficult types of patients to treat, for he persists in his "I am in control" attitude. It is like pulling teeth to get information from him to compile a medical history. However, once he understands the importance of a regime in the treatment of his allergy, he will follow it to the letter. He is self-disciplined. The trick is to make him *feel* in control of his treatment without giving up an inch. The most difficult thing is to get him to change his normal regime to one of avoidance of that which is making him ill.

How did he get this way? He was probably raised by rigid, domineering parents, especially within a family in which the father dominates. They set exceedingly high goals for him and pushed him hard to attain them. They probably planned his life for him.

The Attacker

Dr. Bell describes him thusly:

> The attacker needs to release his hostilities without accepting responsibility or dependence on others. He likes to hit others and to run from obligations. He tears down a plan but offers no solutions. Being an authority rebel, he loves to argue and debate. He is sarcastic, cynical, and negative.

In my office, he's the fellow who states right off the bat, "Look, Doc, you know and I know that this is just going to be a waste of time," or he demands immediately to know exactly what I intend to do. "How can you help me?" he cries, but when I've given him a detailed account of what he must do to control his allergy, it's like rolling Sisyphus' rock up the hill only to watch it plunge to the bottom to get him to follow my prescribed treatment. "Aw, come on Doc, I'm too busy for all that nonsense!" And then he will triumphantly exclaim, "I knew I couldn't be helped! Maybe I ain't even got what you said I got!"

He is the fellow who so frequently says during the first interview, "Look, Doc, I got this little old touch of allergy. Can't walk a block without puffing. What? Stop smoking? Aw, come on, cigarettes never hurt anybody. That's a bunch of baloney and you know it. There's this old fellow I know, see. He's smoked every day of his life, a three pack a day man and he's eighty and still going strong!" Or he accuses, "Aw, my wife probably told you to say that, didn't she? She's been nagging me about smoking like there was no tomorrow!"

How did the attacker get this way? He is, Dr. Bell says, the product of domineering parents like the commander, but rather than being domineering and orderly, the attacker's parents are domineering and inconsistent, rewarding him for a deed one day and punishing him for the same deed the next. They overindulge part of the time, deprive the rest of the time. They are apt to be harsh and treat any signs of independence as rebellion against their authority.

The Avoider

Again, quoting Dr. Bell:

> The avoider needs to avoid failure. His goal in life is to hide. He wants to stay out of trouble. He is dependent on others to lead him. He possesses little self-confidence, and he prefers assignments that are stable and routine. He takes few personal risks and sets low goals for himself.

In my office (he usually comes to me because of eczema), he is apologetic for taking up my time, but he has this skin problem and then there are pains . . . oh, different pains in different places. His wife is with him and he turns to her frequently for confirmation. "That's how it is, right, Mae?" or "Isn't that the way it was?"

I don't know how to say this without being a traitor to my sex, but, so help me, it does seem to be the boy, the man, who is dependent. It seems to me that girls generally have a drive for independence early on. When a mother comes in with her daughter and tries to put in a word during an interview, the daughter will turn on her, scowling, "Aw, you don't know anything about it, Mom!" The dependent son or husband will just sit there. When I direct a question to him, he looks at her expectantly. I can almost see the famous umbilical cord tighten.

The avoider will be quick to assure me, "I'll do anything you say, Doc. Anything to get well! But don't you think I should be drawing workmen's compensation or social security or something? I mean, being disabled and all."

And he will be back soon, saying plaintively, "I did everything you told me, Doc, but that rash is still with me. And I still hurt here and ache there." On close questioning, I find, of course, that he did not follow instructions. Maybe he never will. For he has told me, you see, that he has gone for treatment in the past to Dr. X, Dr. Y, and Dr. Z. None of *them* could help him either!

How did he get this way? Dr. Bell says that while he is overindulged, he is also overprotected. His parents are the worry-worry type that fill the air with imaginary fears, warning of impending doom whenever the youngster tries to do something on his own. They frustrate his independence by scaring the heck out of him and they overprotect by trying to prevent failure in predicting it. Thus, indirectly they rob the youngster of self-confidence. They set low goals for him, inferring that they set a low value on his ability.

The Pleaser

Of this gentleman or lady, Dr. Bell says:

> The pleaser needs to make others like and approve of him. He seeks acceptance from all with whom he associates by being kind and generous and by going along with others, because he would rather make friends than perform a task well. He prefers assignments that involve dealing with people on an easy, sociable basis.

In my office, he is the breezy fellow, all buddy-buddy, with an arm draped across my shoulders. "How'm I doing, Claude?" he'll cry (I never did care much for my first name), or "Hey, ain't you proud I lost two pounds like you told me to?" He's hurt you see, if I don't make a big thing about his loss of weight or because he stopped smoking. He seems to feel that he can buy "good news." "How's the old lungs?" he'll ask. "One hundred percent A-okay, huh?" And then he'll wait for me to brag about those lungs, wait like a child for the held-out lollipop, all eager eyes and smile to please. He is the fellow who likes to be told he has the physical health of a "sixteen year old." If I scold him, "You've got to stop smoking. Now! You've got to stop fooling around and putting it off!" he'll go back to his family doctor and complain, "Why is Dr. Frazier so mean to me. I do everything I can to please him. I did cut down on my smoking." And then, lackaday, the family doctor may give me a call. "You've gotten poor Mr. Smith terribly upset. We've got to reassure him. He's a worrier."

Like the avoider, he has been shopping around for doctors and will be liberal in his complaints. "Dr. M. never tells you anything. He's a doggone sphinx compared to you, Claude. I wanna be told what's wrong with me and what I gotta do." And I may someday get a call from a colleague telling me this patient is complaining that *I* never told him anything!

And while the pleaser may exclaim, "You're the best ol' doc ever!" I will be skeptical, for he constantly seeks approval and benevolence. Treating him is a bit wearing. It sometimes requires uninhibited displays of enthusiasm!

How did he get this way? Like the avoider, he has been overprotected by his parents, his independence stifled. He has not been encouraged to self-reliance, but rather discouraged from moving out of the warm and comfortable family circle. His parents have loved him well, too well in a way, for by smoothing out all the rough places in his path, they have discouraged initiative and encouraged the view that all he needs in life is charm.

The Performer

As Dr. Bell tells us:

> The performer needs to gain prestige and recognition. To do this he maneuvers others and tries to make an impression. He strives diligently to be proper and respectable. Accordingly, he changes his values to go along with the most

advantageous positions, and he is very hard to pin down. He seeks those tasks which maximize his image and prestige, regardless of whether he believes in the tasks.

In my office, he is the patient who misses his desensitization injections because he belongs to so many committees and clubs that he is always dashing from one meeting to another. "I just couldn't make it, Doctor Frazier. The Honorary Sons were meeting that afternoon and, you know, I'm Vice President. *I* had to be there." And on my desk he will park a Very Important book he's happened to bring along to keep his mind occupied out there in the waiting room. The title will be turned in my direction so that I cannot help but notice that this patient of mine is a "brain." He will take pains to tell me in the course of his office visits all about the important job he holds, the great largess he showers upon his little family, the social events he has been attending recently. He will paint a studied portrait of himself for me and go away certain that he has left behind a fearfully impressed physician. It may take him awhile, however, to lose his allergic symptoms. He is just too busy racing around being impressive to follow doctor's orders.

His female counterpart arrives at my office dressed as for a night at the opera or some equivalent social function. She uses cosmetics generously, and is cheerful, happy, animated, gushing. She, too, rides herd on a number of committees and is generous with her husband's money to those who eagerly include her name upon their letterheads.

How do they get that way, he and she? Generally, according to Dr. Bell, they are this way because the parents are "status conscious." The child reflects their own success, so must be pushed and pummeled to succeed, to make his mark, to move in the best of peer circles. But at the same time, the parents are never quite satisfied, and the child soon feels that he never will quite be "somebody." His self-image suffers and so he turns to blowing his own horn loud and long that others might not notice that he is not quite as great as he ought to be. The performer's parents also teach him to skirt the truth a bit rather than to face up to conflict. Thus, he learns early in the game to embellish a bit, to exaggerate. Perhaps in the end he believes it all himself.

The Achiever

Dr. Bell portrays this man or woman as follows:

> The achiever needs to maximize his potential, to reach his highest levels of competence, to become self-fulfilled. He is problem-centered and goal-oriented rather than self-centered, since he has much self-confidence and self-reliance. He works toward challenging, yet realistic goals. He accepts feedback about his results and likes to explore creative new ways to reach his objective. He devotes himself to things he believes in, not those that merely give him prestige or money.

The achiever arrives in my office because he wants to enjoy good health. He will tell me exactly what he has found to be wrong with him, and he will follow my prescriptions faithfully. He will speak and act as if he has faith in my skill as a doctor, and he will cooperate and take responsibility for his own treatment. As a patient he or she is a joy. The achiever will even laugh easily at my jokes, proving beyond a shadow of a doubt that he suffers from no neurosis. In appearance he mirrors his self-confidence and contentedness with himself in his dress. It is odd, but when we say that clothes make the man, we are saying perhaps more than we realize. I have noticed that people who lack confidence in themselves and those with neurotic tendencies are often overdressed, either in an elaborate fashion or studiously casual. Thus, women who appear to have emotional problems often wear a great deal of jewelery and plaster on far too much makeup, whereas men with similar problems will either wear very well-tailored suits and have long fingernails or wear shirts open at the neck to exhibit tanned skin à la Clark Gable or the like. The achiever evidently has no need to project such an image of himself to the world.

So, how did he become such a reasonable, well-balanced individual? The parents of an achiever encouraged independence as his abilities developed. They loved him well and encouraged and supported him in his slow and steady steps toward self-reliance. They gave him responsibility commensurate with his ability and supported him when he failed in such a way as not only to give him the courage to try again but even to enhance his own self-image rather than diminish it. The achiever is the lucky kid, and he knows it.

Once again, these are types. Most of us overlap our personality traits so that we may be part commander, part avoider, part achiever and so forth. Children, especially, will have tentative traits that may or may not end up in the finished adult product, depending in part on their life experiences outside the family circle. You could say, I think, that many infants are tiny performers, cooing and smiling, trying to elicit adult responses of pleasure. A little older, and some are avoiders, clinging to mother and hiding behind her skirts. Boys, especially, may show the colors of the attacker and have to be corralled and held like little calves being branded. The majority of my small allergic patients, I believe, are achievers. They laugh at my jokes and riddles and look me straight in the eye. They make good grades in school and are proud of it. They take their shots with a minimum of fuss; their roars of anguish do not nearly approach my own. They accept a good bit of responsibility for their own avoidance measures (who would not expect some lapses), and frankly I am very proud of them. I hope they know it. I try my best to show them that it is so.

In any case, it's no easy matter to stick labels on human beings. Nor do I believe that it follows that a certain personality type with specific predominate traits will be prone to certain, specific diseases. We tread upon quaking ground when we try to demonstrate that a specific emotional overlay, say, hostility, as indicated by behavior and personality traits is the prime cause for a specific disease such as allergy. We stand a little firmer when we indicate that various diseases can cause specific emotional overlay. Eczema, for instance, can cause a good deal of embarrassment for some; and asthma can cause anxiety when moderately severe.

Let's take an example from the literature of allergy. The emotion of anxiety as stage fright was diagnosed as the cause for an actress's attacks of asthma each time she started to go on stage—until it was discovered that she was extremely allergic to some of the ingredients used in her makeup. Conversely, a man who suffered asthma attacks at dinnertime was considered to be allergic to cooking odors—until it was demonstrated that he became emotionally upset by dinner-table arguments, which precipitated an underlying allergy, probably to food. While we can say, I think, without equivocation that our emotions play a potent role in allergy, to indicate just what that role is takes a modicum of caution.

Now that you are duly warned, come into my office and let's, so to speak, lay on these various concepts of mind and body, emotional stress and personality. Aha, you say, at last you are going to relate this grab bag to allergy? Yes, yes, of course. But wait a minute. Perhaps we'd better make a stab, a brief and cursory one, at understanding what allergy is all about.

7

Allergy Explained

Why John Doe and not me?

That's the question we shall try to answer in this bird's-eye view of allergy. John Doe is our hypothetical allergic patient whose main symptom is asthma. Take a chair over there in the corner out of sight, and I'll fill you in with the details as we go along.

John is our first patient this morning, and he is obviously upset.

"Is it all in my head, Doctor? Do I just imagine I can't breathe or something?" Distressed, he begins to cough, then wheeze. Within minutes his asthma attack is severe enough for me to administer epinephrine. When he is breathing more easily again, I ask, "Why do you think it's all in your head? What makes you believe you can imagine an attack of asthma?"

"My wife," he replies moodily. "She thinks I'm neurotic or something. Even my friends tell me it could be just nerves."

"Well," I murmur as soothingly as I can, "allergy is a rather new medical specialty. A good many people don't understand it, including some doctors. There's much more to it than nervous tension or emotional stress, although they do play a part."

As I compile his "history," the detailed account of his symptoms and background, I discover that John Doe is a prime candidate for allergy. His father had suffered from hay fever, his mother from migraine headaches (some are considered to have an allergic basis). Armed with this allergic inheritance, he, himself, had wandered through a succession of allergy-related illnesses beginning with colic as a baby, switching to eczema when he was about five months old, and arriving now in adulthood at severe asthma. This rather typical progression is often called the "allergic march." John's recollections of childhood are of almost continuous illness, of missing school, of always being behind in his classwork and in the class itself, of not being like other boys, especially after his attacks began when he was about ten years old.

"To put it mildly," he says moodily, "I was a sissy."

By the time John arrived at my door, he had been to several doctors, including an allergist in the northern city where he had lived prior to moving into the Asheville area.

"Dr. X, my allergist up north, told me to stop eating eggs and drinking milk if I wanted to get rid of my asthma. Boy, my mother had a fit. 'Eggs and milk are good for him,' she said. 'They'll make him big and strong,' She swore I'd be a puny wreck, if I didn't starve to death first! But Dr. X was right. It worked. He also treated me for hay fever. Up until he gave me all those shots I used to have to stay in an air-conditioned room all through the ragweed season. I used to hate to see the fall roll around, I can tell you!"

He has, it seems, learned to avoid eggs and milk fairly successfully. This is no easy thing, either, since these two common staples of our daily fare are incorporated into all kinds of food products. He has been successfully desensitized to ragweed pollen and can now venture forth from his air-conditioned hideaway without drastic results. He has also learned, the hard way, to stay away from the close proximity of cats and dogs, since he is also allergic to animal danders, the scales and scurf particles emitted by our furry four-legged friends. He has, in a word, been remarkably successful in controlling his asthma. Until recently.

"I was doing fine," he explains bitterly, "until I got married!"

Oh, come now, you say, getting married surely isn't going to revive a man's asthma?

Hmmmmmmm.

Well, everything has been said about marriage at one time or another, from "Marriage is a necessary evil" to "One was never married, and that's his hell; another is, and that's his plague." Obviously, for John, marriage has turned out to be a plague of sorts.

"Hmmmm. How long did you say you've lived in our area now?"

"About four years. But I tell you, I wasn't having any trouble until six months ago. When I got married. About a month later I began to wheeze again."

"Feather pillows?"

"No! I know better than that. I don't know. My wife thinks all I need to do is buck up and be a man or something," he continues moodily. "Stop worrying so much about yourself, she keeps telling me. She thinks I talk myself into an attack, believe it or not! I guess since she's been as healthy as a horse all her life, and that's exactly how she puts it, Doctor, she doesn't see how anybody can have trouble breathing just because of pollen and such things. She thinks all I need to do is think positively and my asthma will go away."

"You're still avoiding milk and eggs?"

"As much as I can," he replies, resentment raw in his voice. "She thinks it's a lot of trouble to cook without them. She's always complaining about my special diet. Gee, my mother never complained. She was always glad to do something to help me . . . ." His voice trails off and his expression becomes momentarily wistful. I could guess that at the moment he wished himself safely back with Mother.

"And then she's always complaining because she can't have a dog or kitten!" By now, he has worked himself up and his voice is sharp with rancor. "And she thinks I'm just wasting money going to doctors. She got mad when I said I had an appointment with you!"

"Wasn't she aware of your allergy problem before you two got married?"

"Well, maybe not really." He moves over to the defensive now. "You know, I wasn't having any trouble. I didn't think about mentioning it. I guess I figured I was cured or something." He makes a wry face and scratches nervously at the backs of his hands.

The more he talks, the more obvious it seems to me that neither medication nor avoidance measures are going to be quite enough to keep him free of asthma now. He appears deeply depressed, and as he continues, the clues to his emotional state begin to fall thick and fast—like autumn leaves in a rising wind.

Mother, it seems, has played a large role in his life. And still does, as I find out a few days later when she calls me to complain that her daughter-in-law isn't giving her son the proper care. She explains at length that she never could do enough to help him through his asthma attacks as a child, although she waited several years to take him to an allergist in spite of the family doctor's insistence that she do so. But she protected him well throughout childhood and adolescence. Too well. She spun a maternal cocoon around him, and while other children moved step by step out into the world of independence and responsibility, she kept John close, as though the umbilical cord had never been severed. There were many things he was not allowed to do lest they bring on his asthma. Play was severely limited, especially the ordinary rough-and-tumble games of his peers. They, rather naturally, began to look upon him as the sissy he now acknowledges he was. Sports were all but out of the picture. And he did not go away to college because Mother feared he might not be able to take care of himself properly and protect himself against severe asthma attacks. She encouraged him from infancy to follow a sedentary, "safe" way of life. It was all for his own good, she constantly told him. And he adapted to the restraints she set for him by not maturing fully. Now, in manhood, it is obvious that he feels less of a man, less able to cope with adult responsibilities such as marriage. If he resented his mother's continual fussing during his childhood, it seems now to bother him a great deal more that his young wife has made light of the allergy symptoms that brought so much attention and care in the past.

In truth, Jane Doe's view of the matter is a pretty common one. I discover her misconceptions about allergy myself when I talk to her later in my office. It seems that she took several psychology courses in college and was deeply impressed.

"We know, don't we, Dr. Frazier," she begins at once, briskly, "that most of these things are really emotional problems. It's his defense against all the things he can't cope with. Like whenever something comes up at his office he can't handle. Then, too, he uses his asthma to get his way. His mother saw to that, believe me! Why every time something comes up he doesn't want to do—or if I want to go off and do something on my own, painting, for instance, then . . . just then, he begins to wheeze and gasp. His mother would drop everything and rush around to do everything for him. She'd cancel all her plans. She just lives to take care of him! He's always telling me all that she did for him, throwing it up to me! He beats me over the head with the care dear Momma took of him!" Her eyes flash with anger. Clearly, she feels that mother-in-law is prominently at the heart of *her* troubles.

"I just can't believe that if he really wanted to be well, he wouldn't be. If he'd just buck up and take his mind off himself, think of something or somebody else for a change instead of moping about feeling so sorry for himself. I think he finds utility in asthma. I really do, Doctor. Whenever he's upset, he begins to wheeze. His mother just spoiled him rotten!" She flings out that final cry in anger.

Well, there it is. They have let it "all hang out."

What should I do then to set matters right for my patient and, because she is a good part of his problem, for his young wife? Certainly the first thing to do is to make sure both understand the role of emotions in allergy and then what allergy itself is. I begin by drawing them a picture:

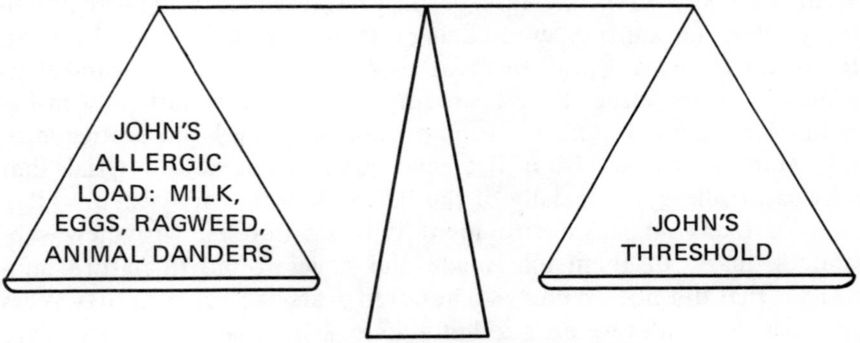

JOHN IN BALANCE: SYMPTOM-FREE

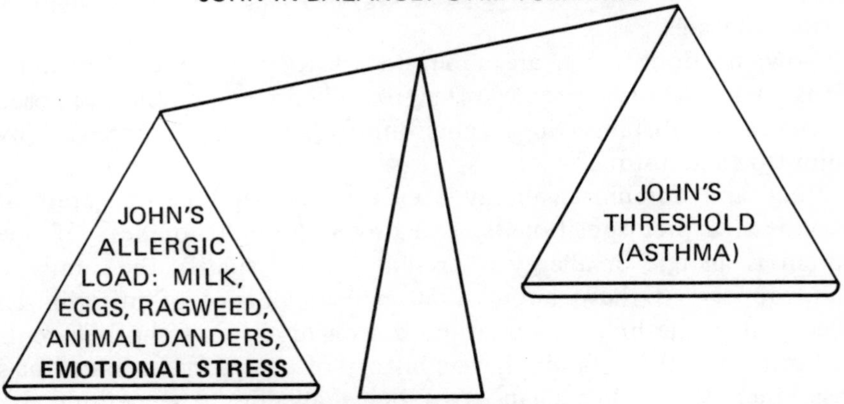

JOHN OUT OF BALANCE
ASTHMA ATTACK!

Now drawing a diagram to explain the concept of the "allergic load" and the individual's threshold is easy compared to explaining just what causes allergy and why. Allergy is a strange business and often does not make sense. So let us take a symbolic deep breath and launch ourselves into the subject.

Allergy is generally defined as an abnormal physical reaction to substances in the environment ordinarily well-tolerated by most people. In John's case, as we have seen, these substances are the very ordinary ones of milk, eggs, ragweed pollen, and animal danders. The majority of us have no problem with such things, but perhaps as many as one out of ten Americans is allergic to one or more things as common as these. In fact, recently allergy has become the number one chronic disease in our nation—a dubious distinction if ever there was one! Statistically, it seems to be still on the increase, perhaps because more and more potentially allergenic substances are being introduced into the food we eat, the water we drink, the air we breathe. A great variety of new and allergenically potent drugs have been employed recently not only in the field of medicine, but also in food production and the cosmetic industry. Many industries also utilize new chemicals and new materials that may cause allergy, especially of the skin and respiratory system. All in all, our technological environment is being flooded with new substances, many of them man-made and never found in nature, substances that did not even exist a hundred years ago—or even fifty years ago. Small wonder we are suddenly discovering that some of them are having an effect on our health—in allergy as well as in other, even more serious illnesses.

Now, no doubt, you are about to ask the most natural of questions. Why do some people suffer from allergy while others exposed to the same substances in the environment are never bothered? Why John Doe and not me?

First and foremost, allergy seems to be an inherited trait or weakness, a predisposition handed down through families. If one parent is allergic or allergy is present on one side of the family, a child appears to have about a 50 percent chance of suffering an allergy to something at sometime during his life. If both parents or both sides of the family have a history of allergy, as in John Doe's case, then the child's chances of being allergic to something rise to 75 percent. Clearly one must choose one's parents with care! However, it must be said also that few of us arrive in this world with a perfect genetic constitution. Most of us have inherited some flaw, some deleterious tendency, large or small, from our doting parents, who, in turn, received it from theirs. The predisposition to allergy seems to be such an unwanted gift from the past. Genetics, then, is one of the main factors determining who will develop allergy disease.

Other factors are involved, however, Almost as, if not as, important as the genetic factor, is the strength of and duration of exposure to allergenic substances. The infant subsisting almost wholly on milk is massively exposed to a potentially allergenic food. That exposure combined with a genetic tendency to allergy is about all he needs to become sensitive to milk. Which is exactly what happened to John. Weather conditions, especially sudden changes of temperature or in barometric pressure, can also be a factor. The presence of infection plays an important role in allergy. Even metabolic and hormonal changes, such as menopause, may make one more vulnerable to the invisible threat of allergens (the label we pin on substances that cause allergy). If we were to redraw the diagram of page 65, it would look something like this:

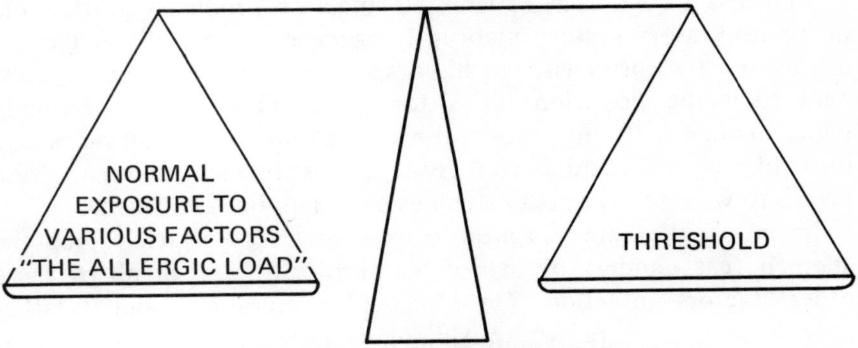

ALLERGY: SYMPTOM-FREE

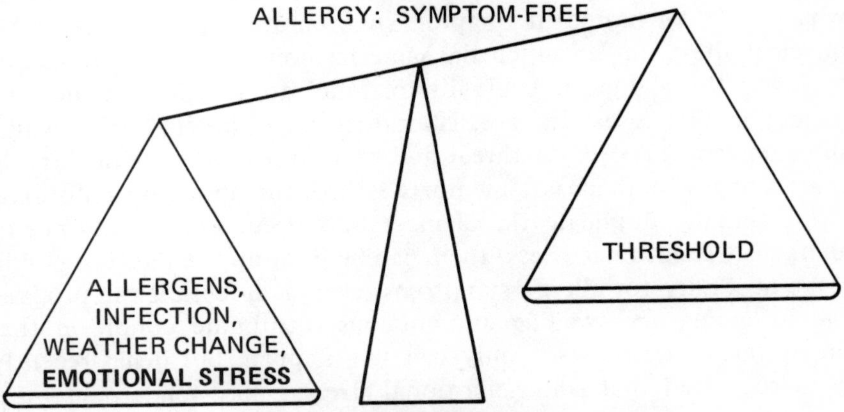

ALLERGY SYMPTOMS

Thus, there is more to the allergic load than one might suspect at first. Small wonder that those who inherit a tendency to a low threshold to allergenic substances get tipped out of balance more easily than those whose thresholds are normally much higher. The greater one's tolerance to such factors, the greater the allergic load must be to broach that tolerance and bring on allergy symptoms. We are not rigidly in balance all of the time. Like finely adjusted scales, we see-saw up and down a little. There are allergists who believe that just about anyone can be made allergic to something at some time in his or her life if factors combine to form a potent enough allergic load. Therefore, Jane Doe should be wary of scoffing at John's symptoms. She, too, could find herself suddenly allergic to something.

If we were to examine John Doe's allergic load on a given occasion, we might find a sequence of events or factors such as the following:

John has a cold. The inflammatory action produced by the cold in his respiratory system is abruptly aggravated when his neighbor's cat makes a surprise visit to his house via an open cellar window. And then the pollution index for sulfur dioxide runs unusually high, further irritating poor John's nasal mucous membranes and bronchi. Now a sudden cold front moves through the area. John begins to wheeze. His asthma comes alive, and he is not well.

In much the same fashion emotional stress of itself plus the allergen (cat dander) or in combination with any or all of these other factors–infection (John's cold), pollution, and weather change–may operate to knock John's precarious balance out of whack. As we noted in Chapter Two, emotional stress can cause physical alterations in much the same fashion as these other factors to lower the allergic individual's tolerance to an allergen, the cat's dander in this case. In fact, laboratory experiments during which subjects were exposed to threat and even to pain have demonstrated that changes in the nasal membranes brought about by emotional stress actually duplicate the changes that occur in the presence of allergens. Emotional stress, then, can help set up the physical conditions necessary for allergy symptoms, even as infection can produce the inflammatory swelling and mucous membrane condition that precipitates allergy. Not only can this happen, but it has recently been suggested that some emotional stresses may tend to suppress our natural immunity or resistance to infections and disease.

Yet, while emotional stress and the above other factors may all be possible adjuncts in John Doe's asthma, they were not, in a sense, direct causes for that asthma. Cat dander was the "cause" of his symptoms. The other factors were "triggers." They precipitated a condition that already existed. If you were to remove the cat dander from the above scenario, these "triggers" or nonspecific factors as they are often called would fail to bring about allergic symptoms in sensitive persons. William C. Deamer, in his chapter, "Environmental Control," in the recent book, *Allergy and Immunology,* edited by Drs. Frederick Speer and Robert J. Dockhorn, illustrated this concept vividly. With his kind permission, I reproduce his diagram here.

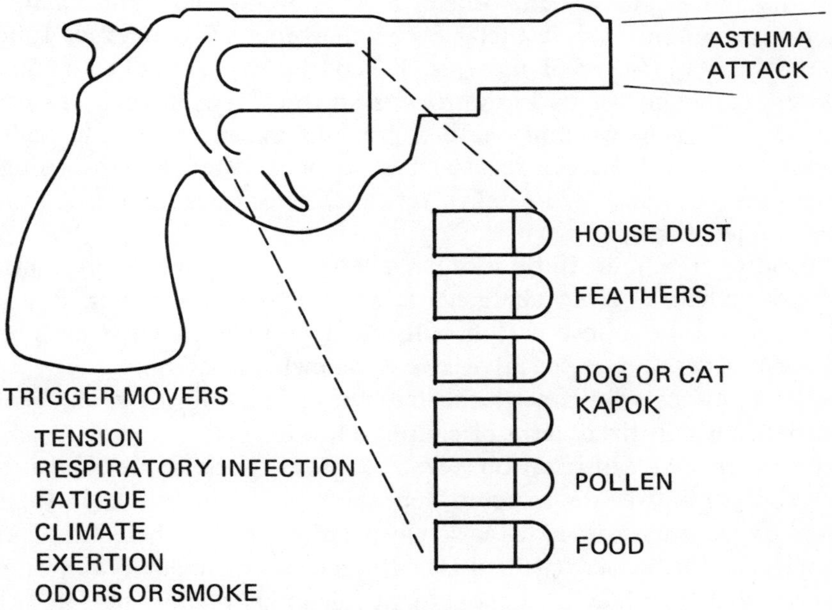

CAUSES OF ASTHMA
ASSUMED VERSUS ACTUAL

Dr. Deamer says:

While the analogy represented here is somewhat oversimplified, it makes the important point that what seems to cause an asthma attack is often only what triggers it, the actual cause being the frequently unrecognized bullet or bullets (i.e., items to which the patient is sensitive). Proof of this concept comes when, following removal of the bullets, the trigger-movers no longer bring on an attack.*

Certainly, not much shooting goes on when there aren't any bullets in the gun. Thus if there were no bullets in the chamber—no allergens of house dust, or feathers, or pollens, or cat and dog dander, and so on—there would be no allergic symptoms. Allergens are a necessary ingredient. They are the primary cause for the physical changes we describe as an allergic reaction. Some of these allergens, such as pollens, we inhale; and some—ragweed pollen, for instance—are more potent than others. Fittingly enough, such allergens are called inhalants. Some we eat (ingestants) and some of these, too, are far more potent than others; milk and chocolate, for example, are more potent than lettuce. Some allergenic substances we touch (contactants). Some of these, such as poison ivy, are apt to be more potent, as many of us know to our sorrow. To become sensitive to any allergen, we must have a previous exposure. Some highly sensitive individuals can react almost at once, after perhaps a single exposure, but usually it takes repeated exposures to bring about allergic reaction.

Route of administration of an allergen has a role to play also. If you inhale a given allergenic substance and react to it, it does not necessarily follow that it will affect you if you eat it or touch it—or vice versa. Our sensitivities are somewhat selective.

Those of us who inherit the tendency, like John Doe, are likely to become sensitized early in childhood. However, many of us may suffer induced sensitization (even without genetic predisposition to allergy) if we are exposed repeatedly to a potent allergen, or even if we are exposed to a single massive dose. There are drugs (aspirin), antibiotics (penicillin), chemicals (formaldehyde), some heavy metals (nickel), the exudants of some plants (poison ivy), and the sting or bite of some insects (bees) that are often responsible for such induced sensitization. Frequently these reactions occur later in life. In a manner of speaking, certain cells of the body "learn" to react to an allergen in this process of sensitization. To illustrate, I had a friend who once attended a PTA meeting

*William C. Deamer, "Environmental Control," in *Allergy and Immunology in Childhood,* eds. Frederick Speer and Robert J. Dockhorn, Springfield, Illinois: Charles C. Thomas, 1973, p. 383.

held in his daughter's classroom. (He claims his wife was especially persuasive this one time in talking him into going.) In any case, he went and sat himself down—not comfortably, I am sure, since he is over six feet tall—at a student's desk and prepared to listen attentively to the proceedings. Somewhere along the line he wished to inject an idea and so, ancient habit once learned and ne're forgot, he dutifully raised his hand like the schoolboy he had once been. The desk, the classroom atmosphere—all combined to bring back earlier learned behavior. Don't smile. Such habits are never easily lost. They reappear in our lives from time to time on cue.

In much the same fashion, once the body "learns" to react to an allergen, once it becomes sensitized as we call this process, allergy symptoms occur upon succeeding exposures to that allergen. Often, too, once the body "learns" to react, it doesn't take much exposure to set off that reaction again. For example, once some people have become sensitive to aspirin, even a crumb of this common household drug may cause allergy symptoms, and for a few highly sensitive souls, aspirin can be a very dangerous thing. It can kill. Body cells, like the humans they compose, frequently learn their lessons quickly and well. Too well on occasion!

An allergic reaction is essentially an immune reaction that's a bit overdone. It's a bit like a helpful Boy Scout who, on rushing to the aid of a little old lady trying to get across a busy boulevard, yanks her across to safety so vigorously that she almost has a heart attack. The body's immune defenses, the antibodies, having "learned" their lessons well, may swarm out to do battle so resolutely with substances they consider as foreign invaders that they damage some of the body's own systems in the process.

But wait, you protest, aren't antibodies supposed to protect us?

True. That would seem to be the grand design. Nothing, however, is perfect. You can have too much of a good thing! An allergic reaction is really overprotection, a too-zealous struggle to repel what are, for the most part and for the majority of us, harmless substances. An overabundance of some antibodies possessed by the allergic individual releases, in this overly energetic struggle, several substances, histamine being one of them, that can actually damage body organs. Where these special antibodies, called Immunoglobin E or IgE for short, are most abundant is where the damage is usually most severe. In John Doe's case, for instance, this happens to be his respiratory system. It could have been his gastrointestinal system, his skin, and perhaps even his central nervous system. These organs of the body that are most vulnerable to such allergic reactions are called the shock organs.

So, if you will hang on to that mental image of the eager Boy Scout doing his duty by pulling and tugging a little old lady at top speed across a busy street, you will have some notion, a picturesque one at any rate, of what goes on in an allergic reaction. It is, of course, somewhat factitious and grossly oversimplified. But, to summarize, the allergic individual probably inherits the tendency to overproduce IgE antibodies. Upon exposure to allergenic substances, and especially upon exposure when other factors such as infection, emotional stress, weather changes, and the like are also present, these antibodies insist upon recognizing these substances as foreign invaders. Once these IgE antibodies have "learned" or become habituated to attack such substances, they do battle with them whenever they arrive in the bloodstream or come in contact with such sensitized or "educated" cells. Just as some of the great monuments of civilization were destroyed during World War II to "save" civilization, so healthy cells are damaged in the IgE antibodies' misguided, if well-intentioned, efforts to save the body from attack.

Combine this situation with the concept of an individual, ever varying threshold of susceptibility to allergens, and you can perhaps understand that in allergy particularly it is necessary to treat the patient as a whole. Causation in allergy is a complex business and follows few rigid rules, at least not to our present knowledge.

There are, in all this, two main types of allergic reaction–immediate and delayed. Immediate reactions include such familiar miseries as hay fever and asthma, eczema and hives. Delayed reactions manifest themselves usually in such discomforts as contact dermatitis, the kind of anguish, for instance, that poison ivy can bring. Immediate reactions may occur within minutes or hours after exposure to an allergen, whereas delayed reactions occur hours or even days later. The main difference in the reactions themselves is that an immediate reaction causes damage to body systems via circulating antibodies, while in a delayed reaction body cells are damaged directly. Because the factor of emotional stress is not a great influence in delayed reactions, and because we will cover the essentials for whatever role it does play in our discussion henceforth, we will turn our attention in the main to immediate reactions.

Oddly enough there is a reverse process to this sensitization mechanism. Called desensitization, it is employed, often successfully, to protect the allergy-prone against some allergens, pollens, for instance, and allergy to insect stings. This procedure works on the theory that repeated exposures to the allergen culprit, beginning with very small amounts and increasing them gradually, can raise the allergic individual's tolerance threshold until he can withstand the onslaught of normal exposure to the allergen in question. However, this process does not seem to work for everybody or for all types of allergens. It has not been very effective in allergy to foods, for example. In addition, for someone who is so hypersensitive that even a minute quantity of an allergenic substance brings reaction, it can be too dangerous to attempt.

What kind of substances are most likely to raise the hackles of IgE antibodies? The list is long, the variety bewildering. Pollen is probably the most widely known villain, but even so, a good many people do not realize that grass and tree pollen can cause the familiar symptoms of hay fever or, more technically, allergic rhinitis. Many are also ignorant of the fact that it is ragweed, not goldenrod that causes so much annual fall misery. Nor are all aware that hay, unless it is moldy (and that is caused by another allergen, the fungi) has nothing to do with hay fever and roses have nothing to do with rose fever. Flowers, like roses, do not depend upon the wind to pollinate, and thus do not scatter their pollens about where sensitive man can intercept them with his nose. It is the inconspicuous plants which rely upon the wind to spread their kind across the landscape that cause so much grief. From early spring until late fall the air is filled with pollens of one kind or another. But pollens aren't the only things we breathe that cause trouble. House dust and fungi are both especially potent allergens and very difficult to avoid. When patients seem to suffer hay fever the year around, the chances are excellent that either or both of these two are the culprits. Then there are such things as cotton and kapok linters being wafted about, arising within the home from aging overstuffed furniture, mattresses, and rugs in the main. And, of course, there's an assortment of pollutants out there either to cause allergy directly or to make us more susceptible.

When it comes to allergens we ingest, the lists can be surprising. Some of our most common foods, the very staples of the good American diet—milk, eggs, wheat, and corn—head the lot. Then there are nuts, fish and shellfish, chocolate, beans and peanuts from the legume family, plus some of the many additives now placed in our food to pep it up, color it prettily, fill it out, smooth it down, or preserve it forever—or, not to exaggerate, for some good while. Pesticide residues and traces of antibiotics and hormones fed to livestock before slaughter can also arrive upon our tables to create their own brand of havoc among allergic persons. The pills we doctors prescribe can sometimes be exceedingly dangerous for the sensitive, and one of the most potent is that old standby of the medicine chest—aspirin. Even some of the dyes used to color medicines can bring untoward results.

For the sensitive, too, the consequences of substances injected can be serious. Bee venom, for instance, can be so powerful an allergen that the sting of one bee can bring death to a hypersensitive individual. A penicillin shot can also result in tragedy, a fact that has been widely disseminated in recent years. Oddly enough, more people die from bee stings than from snakebite!

We are literally surrounded by allergens. We inhale, ingest, or touch them every hour or every day and are sometines injected with them by accident or design. Some, as we have noted, are more potent than others; some affect a great many allergic persons while others cause illness for only a few. Perhaps the wonder is that although we live from birth to death in a veritable sea of allergenic substances, more of us do not suffer from allergy diseases. As a matter of fact, some allergists believe that far more people than is generally realized suffer from "hidden" allergy, a recurrent, generalized feeling of unwellness with vague and diffuse symptoms hard to pin down—or to communicate to a doctor.

So, what kind of allergy diseases and symptoms do these allergens produce? Again the list is long, and while I believe it valuable to reproduce it here, I remind the reader to be wary of that power of suggestion!

The most serious manifestation of allergic reaction is anaphylactic shock, characterized by widespread hives, sneezing, nausea and vomiting, wheezing, signs of weakness, complaints of chest constriction and breathlessness, anxiety, confusion, and collapse. Medical help must be sought immediately, for death can follow.

Such a severe reaction may occur as a result of extreme sensitivity to a drug, usually given by injection, or to an insect sting, but some potent food allergens have been known to bring on this exceedingly serious reaction. It is also thought that some persons hypersensitive to cold may suffer anaphylaxis and perhaps edema of the larynx. It has been suggested that this may explain the occasional and puzzling drowning of otherwise healthy and excellent swimmers.

The role of fear can be so deleterious in this reaction that I instruct my office nurses that they must not act frightened or show fear in any form if confronted by such a situation. It is very important to the welfare of the patient to move swiftly, but to do everything possible not to increase the anxiety of an already badly frightened person. They must go out of their way to reassure him and to demonstrate that everything possible is being done.

Two other kinds of allergic reaction can be potentially serious enough to be emergency situations upon occasion—severe asthma (status asthmaticus) and angioedema (giant swelling) of the larynx area. Asthma can be as frightening as it can be severe, and the more severe the attacks, the greater the anxiety, both for the onlooker and the patient himself. This creates a cycle, for anxiety aggravates the asthmatic attack. Again, medical personnel must not show alarm, but must make every effort to reassure the patient that doctor and/or nurses know what they are about and that he will be all right. Equally frightening is that fortunately rather rare allergic reaction that involves the larynx. Short of such potentially fatal larynx edema, some victims become hoarse and may even lose their voices entirely, sometimes for a long period of time. Such symptoms may be purely allergic in origin, purely emotional, or caused by a virus. Thus, it can present a puzzle for the doctor to sort out. For example, a psychiatrist referred one woman to me because he thought her hoarseness might be due to allergy. We found that he was correct, and we eliminated her problem. It was simply one of the ten miracle cures I limit myself to each day. But unhappily for my standing as a shaman, an almost identical case soon followed which turned out not to have an allergic basis.

Less severe but vexatious are allergic reactions of the gastrointestinal system. Such reactions can pose exasperating and chronic problems for the sufferer and sometimes difficulty in diagnosis for the doctor. We will discuss them at length in a later chapter, so will content ourselves here with noting that our innards often register allergic sensitivities and emotional disturbances, frequently together.

Our skin also is quick to mirror both allergy and emotional stress. There are three general categories of allergic skin problems that we will examine in a forthcoming chapter: Eczema, characterized by intense scratching and a rash; urticaria (hives), characterized by weals and itching; angioedema (giant hives), characterized by swelling. The last is the strangest allergic manifestation of all and can occur in other parts or systems of the body. Many doctors consider it emotional in origin, so much so that in the past it was called angioneurotic edema. Some still cling to that label.

Of course the best-known of all allergic symptoms, as we have noted, is hay fever, more technically known as seasonal allergic rhinitis. Perennial allergic rhinitis, on the other hand, refers to a similar miserable condition that occurs all year around for its victim and is usually the result of sensitivity to house dust, molds, or foods rather than pollens. The role of our emotions in rhinitis is less clear than in asthma and allergic reactions mirrored by the skin, but the role exists.

Finally, and perhaps oddest of all, the nervous system can register allergic reactions. Headaches, motor disorders, and strange behavior may be the result, as we shall see in a later chapter.

Thus, almost any system of the body can be affected by allergy. And as with other illnesses, allergy symptoms can cause fear, anxiety, discomfort, depression. Allergy in itself clearly can bring about emotional stress. Less clear, however, is the reverse proposition—do emotions cause allergy? Are allergy diseases psychosomatic? Other questions to be answered are: Do emotions set the stage for allergy, or does allergy prepare it for emotions? Does a certain personality type react to allergens with a specific allergy disease? Ah well, let's remember with Protagoras, who died four hundred years before Christ, that "there are two sides to every question!"

8

The Allergist as Detective

When confronted by one or more of the bewildering array of symptoms discussed in the preceding chapter, how does the allergist arrive at a diagnosis of, first, allergy and, second, the cause or causes of allergy? How do I know when you, the patient, come to me with complaints of ill health, that you are allergic, and how do I find out just what it is you are allergic to? Do I divine it so to speak, in some magical way? It's nothing so exciting, I'm afraid; but even if the procedure is somewhat prosaic, I do have to work much like a detective solving a crime. Clues are all-important. When I have assembled enough of them, then, it is hoped that I will have the "big picture," all the pieces fitting together to unravel the question of whether you are allergic, and then to what. We must remember in all this that the symptoms of allergy are also symptoms of many other diseases, some of them far more serious than allergy.

The first clues may lie buried in the patient's history. This history-taking procedure, as we have seen, is the initial step for the allergist when a patient arrives at his office. It must be thorough; thus, it may take quite a bit of time and try patience on both sides of the desk. For instance, when you are seated in my very comfortable, leather-padded patient's chair, I try to put you at ease as I begin to question you about your symptoms. What's bothering you? I may ask. After you've reeled off a litany of misery, I may then ask when and where these symptoms occur. Do they appear only at certain times of the year? If so, when? Spring? Summer? Fall? Winter? Any particular hour of the day? Any particular day of the week? Or are they present pretty much all of the time?

This may seem somewhat nonsensical to you, but if your symptoms are seasonal, that's the clue that such allergens as pollen or seasonal foods may be the culprits. If your symptoms occur during all or most of the year, animal dander, molds, house dust, and common foods may be the villains. Time of day may also be a clue, since most pollen is shed by plants early in the morning, while the housewife may stir up house dust, a potent allergen, later in the morning, and so forth. Even the day of the week when symptoms are worse or nonexistent may offer evidence. A man who may be allergic to substances at his office or plant may find himself symptom-free on weekends. Conversely, if something he does at home, mowing the lawn for instance, is causing his problems, weekends may be a time of misery.

We are trying to track down something in your environment that may be causing your allergic reaction: a visit from the neighbor's cat; the acquisition of a new puppy; your wife's energetic spring cleaning; a spell of wet weather that has brought mildew and mold in profusion; a trip into the countryside riotous with ragweed; even the blue-ribbon shrimp plate at your last dining out or the cocktail party where you know you ate more peanuts than were good for you.

So I will go on to ask you if you have noticed whether your symptoms are better at work than at home, or vice versa? Indoors or outdoors? In the city versus country? In your home or the homes of friends or relatives?

I will ask about your bedding. What kind of mattress do you sleep on? What kind of pillows and blankets do you use? Any feathers? Wool? Silk? I will ask about the other furnishings of your house. Have you many books and are they old? Old paper and book bindings can harbor mold. Is your furniture new or old? Again, old furniture with cotton and kapok stuffings harbors mites and mildew and linters in abundance, all highly allergenic.

Are there any pets in the home, even a bird?

Do you know what sort of waxes, insecticides, cleaning powders, and the like are used in your home? Office? Plant or shop?

The "big picture" is beginning to form, but I've only just begun. Now I turn my attention to your daily routine and your diet. What kind of toothpaste and mouthwash, if any, do you use? What kind of soaps, shaving creams, deodorants, and the like? What do you generally have for breakfast? Lunch? Dinner? What sort of foods do you like? Dislike? How much and what kind of liquor do you drink? Do you smoke? If so, how much? Do you take drugs of any kind and for what? Aspirin? Sulfonamides? Antibiotics? Have you ever had any kind of reaction to the latter? Or to any drug?

Hot on the trail, I now turn my attention to the health history of your family, for, as we noted earlier, there appears to be a genetic tendency to allergy. Even though you may have considered the fact that your mother had fierce headaches to be a rather common female failing, the probability is that she was suffering from allergy. Aunt Mabel's frequent colds may simply have been perennial allergic rhinitis, while Uncle Dudley's mysterious rashes may have been eczema brought on by an allergenic food in his diet, such as eggs. Thus, I pay close attention to what went on among your forebears, for it can have some bearing on your own vulnerability to allergy.

And that will bring us to your own health history. I even ask you to go back as far as you can. Do you know whether or not you suffered eczema in infancy? Colic? Did your mother and the family physician have to tinker with your formula? Memory being what it is, I may not be able to extract much helpful information along these lines, but often mothers do keep reiterating to their grown-up children what difficult babies they were, and how hard to please. A colicky baby, for instance, leaves a long and badly scarred memory. In any case, you will surely remember what childhood illnesses you suffered and whether or not you had many colds. You might even know, for mothers are also frequently boastful, whether generally you enjoyed good health and attained normal weight and height ratios and the like. Certainly, you would remember how you did in school and whether you missed much classroom time due to illness. If you did well, you will be satisfied with yourself, and if you did poorly, it is likely still to hurt.

By now, like hounds in full cry after a fox, I am on a hot trail. You have already provided me with a number of excellent clues. Still, we are far from solving the puzzle.

The next step is a thorough physical examination, as much to rule out other possibilities as to rule in allergy. I will pay, rather naturally, particular attention to the organ system that is presenting symptoms. The examination will include lab tests, the most important in detecting the presence of allergy being blood and nose smears. If they indicate the presence of increased eosinophil cells (cells that readily stain pink but are somewhat mysterious in function), allergy becomes an even better suspect. Other tests–such as a chest X ray, urinalysis, a measure of gamma globulin levels in the blood, and blood chemistry studies–are also done, again often to rule out other possibilities; for, as I have said, the symptoms of allergy are also symptoms of many other illnesses, some of them serious. Thus, the allergist-detective keeps an open mind until all the facts are in, but he may have already heard and seen enough to be suspicious. Suspicion, however, is non-science.

When I do tote up the results of this battery of tests, the physical examination, and your history, however, I can say that I believe that sensitivity to something you breathe, eat, drink, or touch is at the root of your problem and that the next step is to find out what that something or somethings is or are.

Some allergenic substances lend themselves to being caught via the procedure of skin testing. However, good diagnostic tool that such testing is, skin tests are not totally reliable. They again are a clue, a piece to take its place in the puzzle. They are most reliable in tracking down sensitivity to pollen, mold, house dust, and other inhalants; but they cannot be counted upon to track down allergy to foods. One exception to this last is that a severe allergy to a food–to eggs, for example–does often show up clearly in skin testing, a fact that sometimes has its own dangers since the aim of the test is to produce a reaction. A severely allergic individual will react to even a tiny bit of allergenic substance–a crumb of aspirin, for instance, or even the smell of eggs being broken open or fried.

Skin tests are simple and not too painful, although the sight of the allergist advancing upon you with his scarificator or hypodermic needle may momentarily dismay. The most frequently employed skin tests are the scratch and/or prick and the intradermal. The first two consist of a tiny scratch or prick being made in the skin, usually on the back or the inner arm below the elbow, into which a drop of an extract of the substance to be tested (ragweed pollen, for instance) is rubbed. In the intradermal test a small amount of the extract is injected just beneath the upper layer of skin. This last method is the most effective in uncovering a weak sensitivity, and is often used in conjunction with the scratch or prick tests after they have given a negative reading, concerning which the allergist is still somewhat suspicious. You would be surprised at how many of these tests we can conduct at one sitting, so to speak. We literally cover the patient's back, keeping track of what drop of extract is where with a cryptic code.

After we have finished decorating you, you then wait for 20 minutes or so to be "read." If nothing or nothing much is produced at the site of prick, scratch, or injection, the reading is negative and you are, at least for the present, not allergic to that particular substance or allergen. However, if a small weal that looks somewhat like a mosquito bite or hive appears and begins to itch a bit, then you are reacting positively to the allergen. Aha! I will exclaim, you are allergic to this. And this! And this! For, you see, commonly when one is allergic to one thing, he is also allergic to other things. Multiple allergies are frequent. For instance, you may be allergic to ragweed pollen, milk and eggs, and poison ivy. You may respond to the ragweed pollen with hay fever and even asthma; you may react to milk and eggs with gastrointestinal distress; and you will, or course, respond to the poison ivy with your skin. However, the milk and eggs can also affect your respiratory system, just to confuse the picture. Allergy to food is frequently the cause of asthma, especially in children. All of which serves to muddy the waters and make things difficult for the allergist-detective. If only you could relate specific symptoms to specific allergens, all would be easy!

You are probably just about to ask me: all right, but if skin testing is not reliable to ferret out an allergy to food, how do you discover what in a patient's diet is causing his symptoms?

Well, when the clues we've assembled so far point toward possible sensitivity to a food, I tell you that what is needed now is an elimination diet. I am aware that you immediately flinch. That word "diet" has become almost equivalent to other four-letter word types in our language. In truth, some allergists are almost sadistic in the diets they prescribe, taking their patients all the way down to spring water and Ry Krisp. And, in order to clear your body of lingering allergens, such a diet must be maintained for 14 to 18 days! If you had meant to shed a pound or two, this sort of spartan regimen will kill two birds with one stone. Some allergists will prescribe four or five foods, all exceedingly nonallergenic (carrots, for instance, and sweet potatoes) during the cleaning-out period. If symptoms continue, they will drop the lot and substitute another four or five. It must be said, however, that these rather grim diets are usually employed only in cases where allergy to food is severe.

More frequently, the elimination diet prescribed simply excludes those foods that are considered potent allergens—milk, eggs, wheat, corn, peanuts, nuts, chocolate, fish and shellfish, berries, citrus fruits, peas; those foods that are suspect from the patient's history; and those foods that show up positive in skin tests, although we would keep a large question mark in mind concerning this last category. If you, the patient, lose your symptoms on such a diet, we then start reintroducing foods one by one, with three- to five-day intervals between each reintroduction to allow you to start up your symptoms again, if you are going to. Of course, if your symptoms return, then we believe we have found at least one food to which you are sensitive. To make sure, however, we remove it from the diet, give your body another chance to clear itself of allergens, and try that food again. If symptoms return, we can then be certain we have found the culprit. In this fashion you will work yourself back to a normal diet with the exception of that food or those foods which bring on your allergy symptoms.

Long drawn-out? Yes, often, but really the only way to go.

Simple? No, not really. There are roadblocks and obstacles to trip us up, and one of them is emotional stress. For example, let us say that you produce symptoms when wheat is returned to your diet, but at the same time you wife has just asked you for a divorce. Now we go around again, give you 14 to 18 days to become clear of the wheat allergens, then try wheat again, but this time your wife has had a change of heart; she didn't really mean it; she was only mad because you forgot the all-important anniversary. So, this time you eat the wheat and produce no symptoms. Thus, your allergy to wheat is mild, and the chances are excellent that you can continue it in your diet, although it would be wise to eat it in moderation and not too frequently. A mild sensitivity to wheat allergens plus anxiety overwhelmed your tolerance. Sudden weather change, infection, or the effects of a second mild sensitivity might also have breached your tolerance to wheat in the same manner.

Thus, like everything else in medicine, elimination diets may not always present clear-cut answers. In general, however, they do produce the villains and, from then on, the rest is up to you, the patient. You will simply have to avoid the food or foods that make you ill. Often such foods are your heart's delight and giving them up can cause real anguish. Be of good cheer, though, for it may not be forever. Often, unless your allergy is severe, in a few months or a year, you will probably find that you can tolerate the allergenic foods if you will eat them in moderation and infrequently. Unhappily, it is often the staple, common items in our diet that can cause the most grief–milk, eggs, wheat, and corn. These are all foods difficult to avoid in our era of pre-prepared and packaged foods. Avoidance requires careful and diligent label reading and some ingenuity in substituting in recipes and the like.

Fortunately, where there is a will, there is a way. The will must be yours after I have provided the way!

Diagnosing allergy takes time and patience. It is not always easy, but I believe it is not nearly as difficult as trying to assess the role of emotional stress in the allergies of my patients. At least I can feel more scientific and every inch the man of medicine as I wield my scarificator and hypodermic needle and shuffle my little bottles of extracts. But the allergist-detective has to move past those allergy symptoms and their allergenic causes to take in the wider horizons of the other factors that can add to the patient's "allergic load," for these factors often make the difference between symptoms and no symptoms. He must be careful to keep the whole patient in view and not become so engrossed in tracking down allergens that he misses clues to these other parts of the puzzle.

Well, perhaps it is time to try to put the various forms of allergy disease–asthma, eczema, perennial rhinitis, gastrointestinal and central nervous system allergy–together with the various emotional stresses alleged to play an important role in their production.

9

The Angry, Anxious Asthmatic

"Doctor, you just don't know the number of nights I sat up with him, watching over him when he had his attacks! The sleep I lost! The heartaches I've gone through because of his asthma! You have no idea what it was like all through his childhood. Even now I worry so . . . . Oh, all the special care and love . . . and then I nearly lost him. But I'd do it all again if I had to. Eddie knows that. I know that he knows I would. I don't mind that he really doesn't appreciate all that I did, all that I had to give up for him. I don't suppose children are ever grateful to their mothers for all that mothers do. I just want him to be happy. To be well and happy. The girls he goes out with, they don't understand. They haven't seen him suffer as I have and held him close, afraid that I was going to lose him. I know that my life was shortened from such worry all the time. And we had to spend so much money, on doctors and such, that now we have very little left. Oh, but that's all right. We were glad to do it to help him and as long as he can be all right now . . . ." Her voice finally trailed off. I cleared my throat, a bit at a loss how to deal with this tirade. Alas, she wasn't through yet.

"All of it will have been worthwile," she cried, "if he's happy and well. But this girl he's serious about, she . . . . Oh, I suppose once she understands his problems, she'll take proper care of him. It's only that she doesn't understand how serious . . . how unwell he is!" Her lips closed firmly; she folded her hands in her lap and stared at me expectantly. I glanced at Eddie. Through all of this, this pale young man had sat there in silence, off to one side, head down, eyes fixed upon the rug at his feet. He did not look up or move, but in the momentary silence I could hear the faint sound of his wheezing.

Well, now, here it was. I was confronted by the classic case of the overprotective mother, the asthmatic son. On my appointment pad, I had marked an office visit for Edward Smith, but evidently Eddie's mother had insisted on coming with her son, a grown man of thirty. So what we have here is obviously asthma and just as obviously emotional imbalance and stress. Is this what asthma is all about? A mother who robs her child of independence and maturity, who wants him dependent upon her and her alone for reasons of her own, coddling and smothering him on the one hand, rejecting him and withholding her affection on the other? Before we try to understand this unhappy situation, we'd better, first, take a brief look at the physical aspects of asthma, then, second, explore some recent thinking on the relationship of emotions to this illness.

The name "asthma" derives from the Greek word meaning to pant or to gasp for breath. This is about as descriptive as you can get. The chief characteristic of asthma is wheezing and breathing difficulties. Not all wheezing is allergic in origin. Other causes may be heart disease, cystic fibrosis, enlargement of the thymus gland in young children, tuberculosis, a foreign object in the bronchus, a malignancy of the lung. However, far and away the most common cause of wheezing is bronchial asthma usually brought on by sensitivity to an allergic substance. This type is called extrinsic, although we must add that there is another type called intrinsic asthma which sports no family history of allergy, no positive skin tests, no increased IgE antibody levels, and no other accompanying allergies. This does not, however, rule out the possibility that it, too, is a reaction to a "hidden" allergy.

And here is where we run into trouble, for there is great complexity and just as great uncertainty in this area. Some allergists have speculated that there are three main kinds of asthma: that caused purely by allergens; that caused by emotions; that in which the two factors coexist. It is more generally agreed, I believe, that asthma that appears before the age of thirty-five is more frequently clearly allergic in origin. After this age, the emotions seem to move in more commonly and take over, so to speak. More about that later. One thing is certain; asthma affects quite a few people. It is estimated that about 5 percent of children under age five suffer asthma to some degree, while about 1 percent of the population at large has asthma. Annually it is the cause of anywhere between 5,000 and 10,000 deaths.

Asthma is obstruction of the airways. The asthma victim's symptoms may begin with a feeling of tightness across the chest or with a dry cough, a kind of continual clearing of the throat. Sometimes, in mild episodes, this may be all there is to it. Or this plus a few wheezes. Fortunately, most asthma patients have mild-to-moderate attacks manifested commonly when exercising or laughing or during temporary emotional upsets. In more severe attacks, however, wheezing becomes increasingly heavy, accompanied by a corresponding increase in shortness of breath. As obstruction in the airways becomes greater during repeated attacks, it becomes more and more difficult to get rid of air trapped in the lungs so that fresh air can be drawn in. During a severe attack, the chest may become distended, and the neck muscles grow rigid in the struggle to expel air. The face may become pale, the nostrils widen, with the posture of the whole body such as to denote the effort to breathe. Often the patient cannot lie down but will sit in a hunched position. His body may become bathed in sweat, and he may soon become exhausted by his struggles. The effort he is making requires the kind of energy one must expend doing heavy labor. The entire scene is extremely distressing for the onlooker and far more so for the patient, who may feel that he is going to suffocate.

What is happening physically to cause such disturbing symptoms? Three main events appear to occur during such an attack. First, chemical mediators such as histamine, released during the allergen-antibody struggle, cause the smooth muscles that are wrapped around the bronchi to constrict, thus narrowing the airways. At the same time, the mucous membranes lining the bronchi swell, further narrowing the air passages. Finally, mucous glands begin to secrete greatly increased amounts of thick sputum which eventually form plugs that not only hinder the inspiration of air but also block expiration. These mucous plugs are nearly always present in the airways of patients who die of asthma, and, once formed, are difficult to treat. The characteristic wheezing sound of the asthma attack is caused by air being forced past these plugs. As if all this were not enough, because the lungs retain an abnormal amount of carbon dioxide, the makeup of blood gases is affected and produces in turn hypoxia, a condition of reduced oxygen in the blood. Such a reduction can affect the heart and brain especially, and at this stage the patient may experience additional symptoms of headache, dizziness, irritability, and an impaired ability to think clearly. Muscles may begin to twitch, the blood pressure rise, the heartbeat increase, and sweat literally pour from the body. The strange thing about all this is that even some patients who suffer such severe attacks may appear to have no disability of any kind in between bouts with asthma. When one has observed his patient literally fighting for every breath of life and then, a few hours later, going about his business as though nothing had happened, it can cause an eerie sense of wonder—even disbelief. Perhaps this is one reason why so many people consider asthma to be more a matter of the mind than of actual physical illness.

Certainly the fact that emotional stress and tension play an important role in asthma is not in question. We express the close realtionship of emotions and the act of breathing: We await revelations of import with bated breath. We sigh in sorrow. Fear takes away our breath, and we hold our breath in moments of danger. We are breathless. A grand view is breathtaking. "Breath," says A. E. Housman in his poem "Reveille," "is a ware that will not keep."

Asthma patients know this above all!

There is one thing that can be said about the asthmatic person: he possesses an excessively irritable or unstable bronchial tract, a condition that predisposes to bronchial constriction. There is a second thing that we can suggest, a theory not yet wholly confirmed: such a patient exhibits an abnormality of the automatic nervous system. This abnormality of function brings about the main feature of an asthma attack, bronchoconstriction. This theory suggests that the asthmatic person's autonomic nervous system is somehow out of balance and abnormally unresponsive in one set of nerve fibers, those that procure the release of epinephrine. Epinephrine, in turn, relaxes the bronchial tract. These particular fibers, the theory proposes, are in some way blockaded, thus leaving those fibers that cause constriction of the bronchi in ascendency. This is a too-simple rendering of a very complex and interesting supposition, and much work still has to be done before all the pieces fall into their proper places. However, if we put together these two possibilities—that an asthma patient possesses an excessively irritable or unstable bronchial tract (and we can probably blame his genetic inheritance in good part for this), and that he may possess malfunction of his autonomic nervous system—we can theorize that he can have two strikes against him at the very least. It would seem then that asthma, whether extrinsic or intrinsic, is based upon a built-in abnormality of one kind or another. Thus we are back to the three general types: asthma that may be caused purely by irritants or allergens (perhaps 3 percent), asthma that may be caused by emotional stress (perhaps 1 percent), and asthma in which both factors play a role. And here I think I will let the matter rest, for much remains unknown, and much is controversial.

It is clear, however, that our emotional life has so far defied accurate scientific analysis (which may be just as well); thus, determining its role in disease is no easy matter. Much of what we know must be based on subjective reports from patients themselves. We can ask them such questions as: How did you feel just before your attack? Were you under the influence of some powerful emotion just preceding your attack? Did you feel anxious? Threatened? Angry? Depressed? And so on. Yet, even after we've compiled stacks of such subjective reports, there is still the problem of individual susceptibility plus the possibility of a number of other factors that must also be considered, such as infection, weather changes, and the like. There are, of course, a number of reasonably (not wholly) objective psychological methods of testing that can be done and the results correlated with asthma symptoms. Even so, the complexity of multiple factors, including the power of suggestion, makes exact determination of the role of emotional stress difficult, given our present knowledge of the brain and body relationship; but all of this doesn't prevent us from taking a crack at it. In any case, I believe that many of my patients are affected by emotional overlay in their asthma attacks.

Let's begin by following the lead of some researchers who divided asthma patients into subgroups, then tried to determine the role of emotions in these groups. For example, one study of children being treated at a residential center for asthma patients separated the youngsters into two divisions: those who rapidly recovered from asthma symptoms when placed under treatment at the center, and those who remained dependent on medication, the powerful steroid drugs, to control their asthma. These were all children whose asthma had remained intractable in the family setting. They had been sent to the center in a process called "parentectomy" (separation from the parents), a sort of last-ditch effort to bring their asthma under control. Surprisingly, some 90 percent of the children so institutionalized for a period of a year or more remain virtually symptom-free. In any case, the results of the above study indicated that the rapid-recoverers had life histories somewhat akin to John Doe's. Mothers were dominant and overprotective on the one hand, rejecting on the other. Fathers tended to be harsh or all but nonexistent in the family. The study suggests that the rapid-recoverers were more influenced in their asthma by the emotional stresses of this sort of family environment than were the steroid-dependent children, whose asthma seemed more truly allergic in nature.

Other studies using subgroupings based on different data such as psychological and personality tests have arrived at somewhat similar results. The rapid-recoverers, incidentally, are the children who most benefit from parentectomy. It can be argued, of course, that removing the child from the family also removes him from the vicinity of allergens that may have been causing his woe. Yet, the surprisingly large number of youngsters who respond favorably to such a step seems to demonstrate that there is more at work in their asthma than allergens. It has been suggested that it is simply a matter of reducing their allergic load by reducing environmental allergens rather than by removing the factor of emotional stress generated in the family setting. To demonstrate that this was not simply the case, at least usually, one researcher employed a novel approach. A group of children whose skin tests showed them sensitive to the house dust of their homes were placed in the hospital. Then dust from the individual homes was collected and scattered liberally in each particular child's hospital room. Almost without exception, none of the youngsters developed asthma symptoms. In another experiment to demonstrate that allergens are not the only villain in asthma, parents of asthmatic children were sent on a subsidized vacation at motels while nurses came in to care for the children. Almost 50 percent of the youngsters improved while Mother and Dad were away.

Thus, perhaps the only really valid criticism of parentectomy is that it may not be permanent. Too often when the children are returned to their home environment, asthma resurfaces. And it is obvious from all this that emotional stress engendered by family relationships must have considerable influence at least on childhood asthma. This has been one of the strongest arguments that asthma, at least some asthma, is psychosomatic in origin. But, whoa, there is yet more to be considered.

Asthma may also be a learned response, a conditioned reflex so to speak. Some asthmatic patients can bring on their symptoms voluntarily by compressing the thorax. The bronchoconstriction thus produced is similar to that brought on by exposure to allergens. It could be then that some asthma begun by allergy may continue on as a conditioned emotional response. This would serve to explain why the asthmatic gentleman allergic to ragweed or whatever has an attack of asthma when shown a picture of the stuff. We are all creatures of habit! But wait, perhaps this is suggestion, as we have noted earlier. Well, if we consider suggestion as a variant of learning, we can have it both ways. In any case, studies in this area have produced some odd results.

For example, in one study that involved 40 subjects, each was monitored by sensitive measuring devices while being exposed to an aerosol saline. It was suggested that this was a precipitant of the allergen to which they were sensitive. About 50 percent of the subjects responded with airway resistance to this nonallergenic substance, a response that was reversed when they were told the aerosol saline was a bronchodilator. It is possible, of course, that anxiety played some part in this experiment. If one suffers moderately severe asthma and has been told he is being deliberately exposed to something that has brought it on in the past, I think he is likely to suffer from some anxiety.

To complicate what is already clearly so complex, we must ask an additional question: why do some people respond to either allergens or emotional stress with asthma rather than with some other syndrome of symptoms or some other body system? We have answered in part: because of an inherited tendency to allergy, and/or a predisposition to an unstable bronchial tract, and/or malfunction of the autonomic nervous system. Asthma becomes the illness of "choice." Thus, emotional stress strikes at an organic weakness or vulnerability—as does allergy.

It has been proposed that suggestion is a secondary factor. An individual especially susceptible to suggestion might, in response to emotional stress, develop asthma because someone in the family or close to him has suffered from asthma or even from wheezing generated by other conditions such as cardiac problems. Asthmatics commonly are afraid of drowning, which isn't so surprising considering that their respiratory tracts fill with secretions. Many a small child whose head has accidentally (or purposely) gone under in a tub or pool has also suffered traumatic fear of drowning. Fear and the symptoms of suffocation may then find themselves joined; and when such a child develops breathing difficulties, say from a bad head cold, you find the ingredient of suggestion for asthma. But again we must note that asthma may start out in response to an infection or allergen as the dominant factor, but be replaced by emotional factors.

What then are the common emotional factors in asthma? We entitled this chapter "The Angry, Anxious Asthmatic" for good reason. Asthma has been called a "suppressed cry" of anger and/or fear of loss of the mother or other sheltering figure. In fact, some asthmatics report that they have abnormal difficulty in crying and that sometimes, when they finally can weep, their asthma symptoms diminish. In this view of the matter, the mother is all-important. If she alternately rejects and smothers the child, she may be indicating her own sense of guilt that she does not love the child as much as she feels she should. The child may sense such lack of love while at the same time he is angered by her overprotection as his struggles for independence are thwarted. One theory proposes that mothers of asthmatic children actually reinforce the child's asthma symptoms to gratify their own emotional needs. Since she could control and dominate the child best when he was ill, such a mother would unconsciously reward his illness with special love and care, whereas when he was well, she might not be so generous with her affection. Thus the child would soon "learn" that to win her love and attention, he needed to manifest asthma symptoms. Yet, in his growing need to be independent as well as loved, the child would be bound to be frustrated. His normal and essential need to become self-sufficient would clash head on with his need for love.

Where is the father in all this? He is absent, ineffective, or not very much concerned about the child.

Do such childhood relationships with the mother explain the psychosomatic aspects of asthma? I don't know. I recently had a patient who suffered a number of severe attacks of asthma following the hospitalization of her grandmother because of a stroke. The patient was clearly anxious. Did her anxiety have its roots in a rejecting and/or overprotective mother? Was the grandmother a surrogate mother? And was my patient overly dependent upon her? Perhaps. But she was also extremely allergic to ragweed pollen, and the season, it happened, was at hand.

Another of my recent cases also illustrates the complexity of determining "cause" in asthma. This patient developed asthma after her nephew burned to death in tragic circumstances. She was distraught and sad, but she also had been cooped up for several days in smoke-filled rooms heavy with the odor of funeral flowers. After the boy was buried and she had returned to her own home, her symptoms diminished. Grief? Or tobacco smoke and flower smells in unaired rooms? Or both?

So, in all this complexity can we single out something so simple as an asthma personality—a specific sort of personality profile, such as one of Dr. Bell's types, who would be the most likely to develop asthma?

We tread on interesting but shaky ground here. This, too, is a matter for controversy. Those who believe that there is a recognizable asthma personality agree that he is a dependent, somewhat immature individual, too much dominated by his mother (or mother substitute, or wife in later years). As a child he is quiet, selfish, and clings to Mother. He pretty much carries these traits into adulthood to become a compulsive, overly neat and tidy, anxious man, lacking in self-confidence and insecure. Quite a bag of traits! According to the proponents of such a profile, he is the fellow who leans on an authority or substitute parent figure, who may be the "do-gooder" who in a very public manner tries to bolster his self-esteem by helping others. He may even, they say, turn out to be something of a daredevil who deliberately courts situations that afford him anxiety. Or he may withdraw into a sort of professional calm, contemplating life from a corner, so to speak. It has also been suggested that he harbors a good bit of hostility and aggressiveness, which he pretty thoroughly represses. He is said to have set high goals for himself and to have had such goals set by his parents, and when he fails to achieve, his already minimal self-assurance suffers badly. He is often deeply depressed.

Aha, you say, I recognize him! That's Dr. Bell's avoider. Or is he a pleaser? Well, whichever, while I find the personality-profile theory somewhat fascinating, I don't really believe such an approach is valid or really very helpful. I think all that can be said is that there is some correlation between some personality traits and disease in general. But I don't believe that there is a specific asthma personality. The traits we can ascribe to the asthmatic person can as easily be ascribed to someone suffering from other chronic and moderately to severely disabling diseases. There is the other side of the coin here—that any such chronic illness can trail enough emotional stresses in its wake to ensure that certain personality traits and/or behavior will be exhibited by a good many of its victims. In many cases I find it difficult to determine which comes first, anxiety and/or anger or asthma—or even dependency and asthma. Certainly illness of long duration is likely to be depressing, its limitations subduing. It would seem highly natural that one's self-confidence would suffer if frequently when one tried to achieve some goal, illness intervened. I am sure that a youngster suffering from moderately severe to severe asthma suffers much the same psychological trauma and personality alteration as one who suffers, say, from a congenital defect that limits his physical and social activity. This is not to say that he cannot be helped both psychologically and physically to live a well-balanced and reasonably healthy life. He can, but it takes more doing than usual and a good bit of common sense on the part of his parents.

The closer we look at this other side of the coin, the more we can wonder whether a given case of asthma can be labeled psychosomatic or somatopsychic (body over mind). For example, in a study of three groups of children—one a group of healthy youngsters, one a group suffering from cardiac disease, and one suffering from asthma—results indicated that the asthmatic and cardiac youngsters both differed in their personality traits from the group of healthy children, but not from each other. Such a finding would seem to refute the specialness of asthma personality possibly. Certainly among the asthmatic group we find some who are much more receptive to emotional factors than are others.

In line with the above discussion is recent speculation that the asthmatic individual has less protection against stress, both emotional and physical, because of reduced adrenal function. Such a theory would appear to place more reliance on physiological, rather than psychological, variation from the norm in asthmatic persons as a factor in their illness. Some interesting studies in *this* area have been conducted at Children's Asthma Research Institute and Hospital in Denver. One study, for instance, demonstrated that lung function among asthmatic children follows a different circadian rhythm than it does among healthy children. The reader will remember that we discussed the importance of biological clocks upon our ability to endure stress. It is theorized that asthma attacks which often occur at night do so because of a decrease not only in adrenal function but in the lung function as well. Experiments with timing steroid (adrenal hormones) therapy to the individual's circadian rhythm indicates that there are optimum times when lesser dosages of these powerful and potentially dangerous drugs can be used to better effect than if the rhythms are ignored. It does appear that we must bend an ear to our own internal ticking, march to our own drummer. It does seem that the asthmatic individuals do not keep in time or step with the rest of us.

If it is true—and I believe that in good part it is—that the emotional disturbances, behavior, and personality characteristics of the asthmatic person are not very different from those aspects that we would find in individuals suffering roughly comparable chronic and debilitating diseases that inhibit normal development and pleasure in life, then the disease state itself has a good bit to do with the individual's personality and emotional distress. Such personality traits that we have just discussed can then be viewed as adaptive, although not necessarily successfully so. Emotional stress then may be as much an outgrowth of disease as a predisposing factor.

The most powerful and potentially damaging emotion in asthma is anxiety. If his asthma is reasonably severe, the sufferer is likely to carry a very real burden of terror. He is afraid of suffocation. Having to struggle for breath *is* frightening. He *is* afraid that he may die during an attack. Unhappily, this fear is all too likely to increase the severity of his struggles, even as continuing anxiety may increase the likelihood of attacks occurring. For when he is symptom-free, anxiety does not necessarily leave him. Alleviating this anxiety may be one of the most important things we can do to help him, but strange as it may seem, I have had mothers of asthmatic children sit here in my office, the child in the chair next to them, and say, "I don't see at times how he will make it through the night!"

Thus, asthma and anxiety tramp around in a vicious circle. Chained to each other, when the one yanks, the other must follow. This analogy, I think, illustrates a good part of the role emotions play in asthma and in allergy as a whole.

It is not surprising then that the asthma patient, beset by his fears, should be more dependent upon others or that he should seek reassurance and security more than healthy persons—the child from his mother, the husband from his wife, and vice versa. The severely asthmatic patient needs a bulwark against fear.

Asthma may also be a physical handicap that can frustrate child and adult alike. The child and the young adult especially may fiercely resent such limitations and may react in one of two ways: by giving up attempts to do and be and withdrawing from the game of life to become passive, introverted, dependent; or by angrily overcompensating to become egotistical, domineering, selfish, hostile, even aggressive. It does not take a child long to discover, for instance, that his asthma can be a weapon to command attention and obedience to his wishes. Nor are adults necessarily immune from such behavior! I have noticed that some of my young patients conveniently begin to wheeze when test or physical education days turn up at school. I have also heard complaints from the wives of some of my older patients that asthmatic husbands tend to wheeze when it's time to mow the grass!

I should illustrate here the problems that face the asthmatic. For instance I had a young seven-year-old male patient whose asthma was well controlled until he went to school. He was obviously a nervous little boy with a slight stutter. He got into a fight with his peers, perhaps over being teased for that stutter. According to the teacher, the youngster "got furiously mad at the other children and lost all control." He also got considerably overheated. The upshot? Eight days in the hospital with asthma. That's hard lines for a growing boy. It's normal enough to get into a fight and normal enough to get "furiously mad," but to pay for it with eight hospital days of asthma is pretty rough.

I treated another youngster recently, a ten-year-old girl from a very poor family. She had suffered wheezing spells off and on for a year, but when her half-brother took to the bottle with all that that might mean in family disruption, the child became very upset and had to be rushed to the emergency room of the hospital for treatment of severe asthma.

Another youngster, a boy of twelve, is brought to me periodically by his very commanding mother. Whenever he tries to say something to me, she snaps at him to shut up. He immediately stops talking and sits quietly, usually staring at his hands in his lap or off into space with a vacant gaze. Mother is so involved in his asthma that she brings in a thick file each visit of all the experiences the boy has had and all the things he has done since the last visit. He must often feel that she is a paid-up CIA agent or a household member of the FBI!

I hope these brief illustrations portray the close interdependence of emotions and asthma and asthma and emotions. I suppose that how deeply personality traits become graven in the individual depends rather naturally on the severity and duration of his asthma, plus the kind of family and social support he receives—or the lack of it! And how chronic illness of any kind, not just asthma, is handled in the child is all-important to the adult personality as well as to the child's. If the child learns to use illness as a weapon or as a passport to his heart's desire, there is little reason why he will not continue to do so as an adult. But most probably he will do so with diminishing success, since the cold, cruel world takes a dim view of immaturity and irresponsibility. Unfortunately, once such an unhealthy habit is established, it's not easily set aside. Once the asthmatic individual passes through childhood's door, his bag of inappropriate responses on his shoulder, he will need all the help he can get to adapt to the real world with healthy behavior rather than disease. Since children are experts at this kind of gamesmanship, parents must be wary not to reinforce or condition the aspects of the child's personality that they may not wish to see in the grown-up product. As has been often stated on all kinds of authority, our ability to handle the stresses of adult life is largely determined during our earliest years.

10

A Cold? Or Allergy?

We stood watching, my friend and I, as his Brittany spaniel sneezed again and again, so violently that he banged his nose on the ground. Between sneezes he would look up at us with a puzzled expression. Suddenly he began to paw at his muzzle, then threw himself into the grass to shove his head about, snuffling and sneezing the while.

"What in tarnation ails him?" my friend cried, alarmed.

"He's got hay fever, I imagine."

"Hay fever? Aw, come on, Claude! You allergists see pollen behind every bush!"

"On every bush," I corrected. "Look over there, at the edge of the meadow. That's ragweed, right? And your dog just came from over there, didn't he?"

"You've got to be kidding! My dog's allergic to ragweed?"

"Could be. I once read about a whole dairy herd that suffered from hay fever because of all the lush ragweed in their pasture. You can imagine that, can't you? A whole herd of sneezing, sniffling cows!

My friend stared at me, truly awed. A thought flitted through my mind. Maybe I could develop a sideline–allergy shaman for the animal kingdom. However, I had to dismiss it quickly, for I happen to be allergic to animal dander. What could be worse than a sneezing, snuffling herd of cows would be a sneezing, snuffling allergist trying to attend to their ills!

For humans, you see, all this is really not an amusing matter. Although hay fever is a nuisance and a misery, at least it has its seasons and is gone. But the victim of perennial allergic rhinitis may suffer much the same symptoms off and on all year round, and such a chronic condition often moves on to asthma.

Quite seriously, our nasal structures not only serve to protect our inner world by sifting out potentially damaging substances from the environment, but they are also extremely sensitive to a number of things–viruses and bacteria, allergens, strong fumes, odors, dust, fungi. The mucous membranes of the nose even respond to drugs ingested or injected and to allergenic foods that do not come in contact with the nasal structures themselves. When we do "follow our noses," they are in a somewhat exposed position.

The nose is a shock organ and as such responds to the antibody-allergen battle by swelling and an overproduction of secretions, but the eyes and nasopharynx may also be affected. Hay fever, which is not caused by hay and rarely if ever sports a fever, is technically known as seasonal allergic rhinitis or pollinosis. Its nasal look-alike, perennial allergic rhinitis occurs, as we have noted, on a chronic, any-time-of-the-year basis. Symptoms of hay fever and perennial rhinitis are often itching nose; itching, watering eyes; a feeling of stuffiness; headache; coughing (especially at night)–symptoms that seem like those of the common cold but are not. Because hay fever sufferers are legion in the United States, numbering perhaps as much as 10 percent of the population (plus some assorted household pets and dairy cows), this particular misery is well known and reasonably well understood by most people. We probably all know at least one person who has come to dread the warm and airy breezes of late spring, full summer, and early fall when the air is full of grass, tree, and weed pollen, when even in the heart of Manhattan the pollen count runs high, when clouds of the stuff drift over the land and far out to sea, when yellow rafts of it float about on rivers and lakes. Victims may never have seen a bale of hay, may not even know what hay is good for, yet suffer all the same. One hundred fifty years ago it was thought that the sun's rays caused hay fever, since symptoms sprouted during the sunny time of year. Some thought heat was the cause, or simply the smell of grass. We know better now, but we are still somewhat uncertain why some of us at some stage of our lives suddenly become sensitive to pollens while the rest of us live and die scot-free; or why some who do become sensitive, do so to some pollens and not others. We know that infection, weather, and genetic vulnerability may have something to do with who gets what. And, of course, to some extent emotional stress plays its mysterious role. Of all the allergic illnesses, hay fever appears most clearly a response to a specific allergen or allergens. As for emotions, while we have the story of the lady shown a paper rose that looked so real she immediately responded with hay fever symptoms, emotional stress probably plays a lesser role in this illness than in most other allergies. However, I must point out that one famous allergist described a patient who began to sneeze during the garden scene in the opera *Faust!* In the main, however, I think the emotional distress of hay fever victims is a result of the condition itself. The sheer nuisance of the thing should account for a good bit of irritability and depression, for instance.

Perennial rhinitis has a much greater relationship to emotions, so much so that some allergists differentiate what they consider a clearly allergic nonseasonal rhinitis from a vasomotor rhinitis for which no specific allergen can be discovered and which may be due to irritating fumes, extreme cold or heat, even looking up into a bright sun, and emotional factors such as anger. In the first instance, molds, house dust, animal dander, feathers, and foods are the more common allergens. In the case of foods, perennial rhinitis may take on the appearance of hay fever when the allergen at fault is a seasonal food such as strawberries or melons. A good many people who suffer from perennial allergic rhinitis also suffer hay fever, which seems like double jeopardy.

To illustrate the role of emotions in each form of rhinitis, let's look at the problems of two ladies. Mary Smith came to me several years ago for help with her hay fever. Her family history spoke of allergy, for her mother suffered both hay fever and asthma and a younger sister suffered from on-again, off-again eczema. When skin-tested, Mary was found to be sensitive to ragweed pollen. Oddly enough, she had learned from painful experience that she could not drink milk during the ragweed pollen season without also suffering gastrointestinal symptoms and a worsening of her hay fever. During the rest of the year she could drink milk with pleasure. The reason? She was also mildly sensitive to milk so that when she was carrying an allergic load of ragweed pollen, her threshold for milk allergens was lowered, resulting in symptoms of allergy of the gastrointestinal tract in combination with hay fever. When her allergic load was light during the rest of the year, she had no problems with milk. Her threshold remained reasonably high, a barrier, so to speak, against symptoms.

As for emotional stress, Mary's problems seemed to begin and end with her streaming eyes, her obstructed nose, her paroxysms of sneezing.

"I just hate to go out of the house when I'm like this," she muttered, swiping at her eyes and nose with a fistfull of Kleenex. "I hate to go to work in the morning. Everyone turns to look at me, I'm so puffy and teary. And at work I make an awful pest of myself, I know. I sneeze until quitting time, and I'm sure it doesn't go over big with the customers. Have you ever tried shoes on somebody, Doctor, while you're having a sneezing fit? Not to mention constantly sniffling or having to go for your Kleenex. It's embarrassing and it's darned depressing."

That she was depressed, irritable, and unhappy was obvious. Just as obvious was the loss of these emotions once she had passed through the desensitization process and could face ragweed season with scarcely a sneeze. As long as she kept up her precautionary shots before ragweed pollen season began, and refrained from drinking milk for a few weeks, she was symptom-free. And depression and irritability vanished, along with her embarrassment.

Susie Jones, however, even though she sported similar symptoms—streaming, itching eyes; runny, obstructed nose; swollen mucous membranes—presented me with a case as different as chalk from cheese. Susie was a housewife, albeit a recent housewife, for up until a year or so earlier she had been remarkably successful as a big-city interior decorator. She made a high-bracket salary and her services were much in demand. Then one day she fell in love, got married, and gave up her career at her husband's insistence. Being somewhat prosaic, he did not wish his wife to bring home more money than he did. Besides, he looked forward to home-cooked meals, the kind his mother used to dish up.

"I loved my work," Susie told me wistfully. "But I could see how it hurt him that I earned so much more. But, Dr. Frazier, I'm so bored, I could scream! I hate housework, but it would be a blessing if there was enough of it to keep me busy. With a two-room apartment, I've done everything I can think to do by eleven in the morning. Anyway, it's the same thing every day, day in and day out. There's not a shred of challenge. I don't even like to cook or I'd go off and learn to be a gourmet cook or something. Oh, I want so badly to get back into my old job that I dream of layouts at night. And materials and colors! I work all night in my sleep matching rugs and drapes and . . . well, you know?" She twisted her hands in her lap and sighed, the very image of boredom and frustration.

"And now," she added almost wailing, "here I am with this awful stuffy nose and postnasal drip and weepy eyes! It's just too much!"

Aha, you say, housewife's syndrome!

In a way, you may be right. Actually, Susie didn't "shop" around for her "out" by consciously choosing rhinitis, for it turned out that she skin-tested as being sensitive to house dust. Perhaps a lucky break for her.

Well, you say, with a hint of impatience, did her boredom and frustration bring on her allergy?

I shrug a little, as shamans often do. Let's say that Susie was predisposed to allergy, perhaps genetically, and she became sensitized after her contact with considerable house dust. Boredom and frustration undoubtedly accentuated her allergic load. There was a "bullet" all right, the allergen of house dust, but there was also a "trigger," her conflict of being trapped between her pleasure in her career and her love for her husband. I think that we can say without quibble that emotional stress was a large factor in her rhinitis symptoms, but I don't think we can say it was the prime cause.

Once again, it's odd how we express in our language the relationship of emotions with our various physical parts. We speak about "paying through the nose," indicating that it's going to be painful. We accuse someone of having his "nose out of joint," implying that there is envy and hostility involved. The nose is a sensitive instrument. It registers grief, prickles with anger, sniffs out trouble, and, according to some researchers, records sexual excitement. Nasal responses vary a great deal among individuals and from time to time for the same individual. Congestion and overproduction of secretions in such nasal responses seems to be a defense mechanism, a kind of "shutting out and washing away" process. It is the mechanism by which we attempt to shut out noxious substances in the environment and by which we weep away our grief and anger. But when this response is prolonged, it can produce pain, discomfort, illness.

One very interesting study demonstrated clearly how this nasal response can occur in reaction to a number of quite different stimuli. When subjects were exposed to the irritating fumes of ammonium carbonate, their nasal passages quickly swelled and produced copius secretions. The mucous membranes became inflamed and reddened, and the subjects commonly suffered also from watering eyes and coughing. Their noses did their best to "shut out and wash away" the penetrating fumes. Such a defense mechanism was also demonstrated initially by subjects exposed to pollens to which they were allergic, although the mucous membranes in this allergic reaction soon changed from red to a pale grayish color. In any case, the nasal obstruction and secretions seemed as clearly a defense mechanism as against the fumes of ammonium carbonate. Perhaps the hay fever victim would like to accept this view of what can be such a nuisance. The idea that he is defending himself annually against the onslaught of the best that the plant world can throw at him may not only provide him with new insight but make him feel somewhat like a sturdy warrior repelling an attack upon the castle!

However, the investigators in this study were not done with their volunteer victims yet. Fiendishly, they rigged up a sort of medieval torture instrument to induce severe headaches. This mechanism, a sort of steel crown that was gradually tightened, was not only unpleasant but represented a threat and thus produced anxiety in the subject. Lo and behold, both eyes and nose went through the same defense maneuvers of "shutting out and washing away." Pain, then, could be added to the list of stimuli that would produce this response in the nasal structures.

Then, in one final experiment, the researchers attempted to see what pure emotional stress would do. They reminded one susceptible subject whose nose was operating normally at the time about certain features of his exceedingly unhappy marriage, thus generating considerable emotional stress. His nasal structures immediately responded in the classic manner, with obstruction and secretion. The investigators suggest that even verbal threat can give rise to this defense mechanism.

Some students of this mechanism suggest that it arises in infancy and becomes a conditioned reflex to be carried throughout life. Certainly we arrive in this world with a cry and often begin to weep with our first breaths. I suppose you could say that we come already on the defensive! The infant wails, seeking gratification and love from his mother. So, it is suggested, do those who respond to emotional stress with their noses. Men in particular, it is said, who are denied the comfort of open weeping in our culture, may respond to frustration or depression with rhinitis, a "respectable" outlet for their distress.

So, is there a rhinitis personality profile? Those who say yes suggest that he is much like their asthma personality—a dependent individual of low self-confidence who turns a somewhat nervous aspect to the world. He is, they say, apt to be in conflict, struggling perhaps with guilt, anxiety, resentment, anger, hostility, or frustration. It would certainly make my life simpler if I could diagnose my patients simply by the personality traits they exhibited. However, in my own lengthening medical experience I haven't yet found that personality X equals disease Y. I believe that the emotional stresses that do color our personalities must take their place with other factors that play a large role in perennial rhinitis, allergic or otherwise—such things as weather, infection, air pollution, allergens, and the like.

To rush back to the role of emotions in what is clearly allergic rhinitis, let me quote from the letter of a very perceptive woman, Mrs. Karen Webster, Home Economics Specialist with the Department of Agriculture, Province of Manitoba, Canada. Mrs. Webster writes:

> I suffer allergic reactions to a lot of things but particularly molds, dust of all kinds and cigarette smoke. I certainly don't consider myself incapacitated by the allergy, although a runny nose and some wheezing, at times, is uncomfortable and embarrassing. For a long time I've felt emotions and fatigue have something to do with *how* allergic I am. For example, if I am apprehensive about a social affair—don't know all the people, not sure of the etiquette for the occasion, etc., my reaction to smoke seems to be more severe than if I am more comfortable in the situation. I will very often start wheezing in this case (mild asthma here, I presume). Also, at work, if I am under pressure with a lot of public meetings scheduled or evening work, I find I tend to be more allergic—from fatigue or emotional stress or both.
>
> Lately, however, I seem to be able to exert some control over this. If I acknowledge to myself that I'm going to be in a smoky situation or find myself in a smoky situation, for example—I find if I concentrate on relaxing or on breathing slower I sometimes have no allergic reaction whatsoever. Sometimes,

> after initially concentrating on relaxing, I forget about it but still seem to be free of a severe reaction. Also, just lately I have been under pressure at work and I knew I was going to. Before and during this period I concentrated on relaxing between work periods, got enough sleep, etc., and although I had more allergy reaction than usual, it was not severe and I wasn't kept from sleeping by wheezing.
>
> This is really interesting to me because I have been led to believe, by various medical people, that emotions were not a factor in allergic reaction!

Oh, yes, they are!—as we are diligently trying to illustrate here. And, thanks to Mrs. Webster's letter, we have added another nail in our structure. One of the great things about writing this book has been the response of people all over the country to my requests, printed in all sorts of journals and magazines, for information and personal experiences with allergy. Fellow doctors and laymen alike have written me letters about their own experiences and those of some of their patients and/or have sent clippings and articles dealing with our subject. I am immensely grateful for all their help. I would like to share all of it with the reader if only space permitted. That is not the case, however; so I will have to pick and choose. For example, here is an interesting letter that describes an opposing view of the situation from that of Mrs. Webster. This letter from Don Savage of Jamison, Pennsylvania, somewhat parallels Susie Jones's problem discussed earlier in the chapter.

> My experience has been that allergies occur during periods in my life that are peaceful, calm and uneventful or non-emotional. [Boredom?] At the first sign of any allergy (running nose, eyes watering), I do something exciting and the symptoms leave *immediately*.
>
> I also have some control over the adrenal gland, and a shot or adrenalin dump will immediately clear the allergy. So that, for example, driving my sport car fast, playing loud, exciting music, will usually do the trick.

Mr. Savage has something here, for epinephrine (adrenalin) is the drug of choice in many cases of asthma because it relaxes bronchospasm. I suppose we can ask whether boredom, perhaps even frustration of mind and spirit, elicits allergy symptoms, while excitement, either because it does spur adrenal gland function or simply because it occupies the mind, relieves allergy symptoms. Perhaps all we need to say is, if it works, fine!

Another letter, from William Hallahan of the Zoology Department at Duke University, enlarges on Mrs. Webster's observations and echoes Mr. Savage:

> My most pronounced allergic response is complete obstruction of my nasal passages to the passage of air. I have found that not only can my emotional state influence the allergic response, but the allergic response can influence my emotional state. For example, small spaces without access to fresh air (e.g., elevators, airplanes, apartments) often cause an allergic response, which in turn creates a feeling of claustrophobia. In addition, situations involving frustration are particularly effective in eliciting an allergic response. For example, if I am working on some project that is initially running smoothly, but suddenly I reach an impasse (due to some mechanical failure), I often have my nose close up immediately. On the other hand, excitement or physical exertion invariably clears up a stuffy nose.

Several illustrations from my own practice may help shed light on the role of emotional stress in perennial allergic rhinitis. For instance, if we are fortunate enough to live long enough, we face the rather extreme life change of retirement. A good deal has been written about what this may mean to a husband put out to pasture, but not nearly as much attention has been paid to the sort of stresses his retirement may place upon his wife. I have recently treated a patient who was fine until her husband retired several years ago. She then began to suffer allergy symptoms, especially a runny, congested nose. She says that her husband has continually complained, growled, and griped since he left his job, and she is very much aware that anxiety brings on her nasal response. In fact, when her husband became suicidal, she had a bad flare-up of her symptoms. Her hope, and mine, is that her husband will soon adjust to retirement.

Another patient of mine who admits to being a perfectionist of sorts has noticed that eye irritation and nasal congestion become more pronounced when she gets involved in a good bit of church work and attends quite a few meetings. She says that she gets keyed up and wants everything to be just right. Most of her work begins in the late fall, and she has noticed that year after year, her allergy symptoms get worse at the same time. This last fall, she worked on a very involved project that required a good deal of planning, phone calls, meetings, and the like. The result? Her symptoms were far worse than usual!

A good many of my colleagues in Ear, Nose and Throat practice believe that nasal erectile tissue does respond to emotions–anxiety, hostility, frustration especially. Add a similar response to allergens, and you have double trouble!

On the other side of the coin, of course, are the emotional stresses that both hay fever and perennial allergic rhinitis trail in their wake. Mary Smith, attempting to try on shoes for customers with a fistful of Kleenex in one hand is a case in point. The youngster in a crowded classroom told to stop his incessant sniffling "right now!" is sure to feel humiliated and embarrassed. Worse still, he's apt to be nicknamed "Rabbit Nose" because of his constant facial contortions as he tries to clear his stuffy nose. He may also have picked up the very noticeable habit of the "allergic salute," a distinctive sort of wiping of the nose with an upward movement of the palm of the hand that is often employed by youngsters trying to ease their nasal obstruction. In time, such a habit may leave an equally distinctive crease across the bridge of the nose. He may even pick at his nose nervously in an attempt to relieve the feeling of being blocked up. Parents and teachers alike will no doubt harshly jump on this habit, creating further embarrassment. Often, too, since his nose is a poor instrument for getting air to his lungs, he may take to mouth breathing. Few parents care to see their handsome, charming child begin to resemble the popular conception of the village idiot. "For heaven's sake, shut your mouth!" "Look out, son, a fly with fly in!" And so forth. Nor for an adult are streaming eyes, a constant sniffle, and loud paroxysms of sneezing social assets likely to impress and endear. Anyone who has ever sneezed repeatedly during a church service will have an idea of the allergic rhinitis victims' feelings–as will anyone who has suffered a sniffle that would not be stifled in the quiet of a crowded library!

All this may be a little on the facetious side, but there really are emotional concomitants to allergic rhinitis, seasonal and perennial.

Before we take leave of the nose and respiratory allergy in general, we should note some recent findings that suggest that surgery with general anesthesia in youngsters under two years of age may predispose to major respiratory allergy. In one study of infants and very young children operated on for pyloric stenosis (an excessive thickening of the muscle at the opening between the stomach and duodenum that causes constant vomiting, constipation, and failure to thrive), some 53 percent later developed allergy disease. Some 45 percent of very young children operated on for hernia later developed respiratory allergy. Another study, of 1,200 homes with children under eighteen, turned up these results: (1) of the allergic children in these homes, 11.6 percent had been hospitalized and 6.4 percent anesthetized; (2) of the nonallergic, 7.2 percent had been hospitalized and 2.6 percent anesthetized; (3) the incidence of allergy in boys who had been hospitalized and anesthetized under the age of two was 35.1 percent. Did the emotional trauma of surgery predispose to allergy? Or did the physical insult of anesthesia? At the moment, no one is sure.

Another recent theory has been developed from a study of a group of children suffering from allergic rhinitis compared to a similar group of nonallergic youngsters. Significant growth retardation was found among the allergic group as compared to the growth records of the nonallergic. If this at present speculative finding proves to be valid, we can theorize that growth retardation among allergic youngsters might also generate emotional stress to further aggravate their illness—not to mention personality traits!

Allergy, which was considered a sort of medical fad 10 or 20 years ago, is now expanding its scientific boundaries. Both new theories and new findings are being announced in rapid-fire fashion. It is difficult for even an allergist to keep up with them, not to mention the general practitioner. And in spite of everything we know today, the sheer complexity of multifarious factors contributing to cause and effect in allergic disease makes definitive statements a bit iffy, especially when we try to pin down a patient's subjective emotions. As an allergist, I often feel that I am really asking for the equivalent of an Augean stable to muck out or a Herculean Knot to untie.

For example, one of the latterday problems I face is to get my rhinitis and asthma patients to stop smoking. I am sure that a heavy smoker already has an emotional problem, and I also know that unless he quits, he is going to have a continuing allergic problem, not to mention other health hazards such as emphysema and lung cancer. Now it's not easy to break the smoking habit as a good many of you out there know. But I am very firm. "Cut it out!" I say. "Don't just cut it down!" I even accuse my more obstinate patients of being unfaithful to me. "Aw, come on, Doc, how so?"

they ask. "I'm cutting down, aren't I? What more do you want?" So I thunder, "And if you told your wife just after your marriage that you were cutting down on seeing your old girl friends, what would she call it?" By then, such patients usually look sheepish. At least so I hope.

I do try hard on smoking. Recent findings have made it imperative for my allergy patients to kick the habit. So, while I rant and rave, I do more. I am unstinting in my praise when they do quit. In front of such an exemplary patient, I dictate a letter to his referring doctor declaring this wonderful news. I walk to the front desk with him, my arm draped around his shoulder, and loudly proclaim his courage, his willpower. This behavior may be classified as shamanship, but it's no act. I am genuinely happy and genuinely proud of him. All on his own he has taken a giant stride to restore his own good health and, for that matter, emotional maturity. I cannot praise him enough. I even keep a book that began with blank pages but is now rapidly filling up with names of those heroes who have stayed away from cigarettes for six months.

Thus, you can see an allergist, besides trying to keep abreast of all that is new, and an awful lot is, must also be all things to all patients and employ his own brand of psychology, or if you prefer, witchcraft, as we shall see in greater detail in later chapters.

11

What the Human Skin Can Register

"Now, Claude, I suppose you're going to tell me that that dog has an allergy?" my friend remarked sarcastically, pointing to a large poodle busily scratching himself beside the curb.

"That's right," I replied laconically in my best Sherlock Holmes manner.

"Oh, come on, Claude," my friend cried in exasperation. "Dogs have fleas. Fleas bite. Dogs scratch. It's as simple as that!"

"True. But dogs also have eczema quite often I'm told. Eczema itches. Dogs scratch."

My friend stopped dead in the middle of the sidewalk, his face expressive of pure disbelief. "Now I suppose you're going to tell me all about a herd of dairy cows with eczema, too! Like that bunch of sneezing, sniffling cows you told me of the other day!"

"Hmmmmm. Now that you mention it, cows do get hives. From being allergic to their own milk. But I suppose you'll find that difficult to believe, won't you?"

"Ah, Claude, Claude," my friend said pityingly, and we resumed our stroll.

But, you know, I'm right. Dogs do get eczema. Cows do have hives. Human beings have both. In fact we humans can produce a nice variety of conditions upon our hides. For all kinds of reasons. Some of these conditions are mainly allergic in origin, some are mainly emotional, but many are probably a goodly combination of both factors.

We present ourselves to the world clothed in our skin. While our hide may not be exactly the mirror of our souls, it does tend to reflect in good part the physical and emotional disorders of body and mind—both fleeting and long-term. Any shaman worth his gourd rattle knows this well! And again, if the reader will but contemplate a moment, he will find our language reflecting this idea. "Don't be so thick-skinned!" we say, meaning don't be so insensitive. "By the skin of his teeth," we say, meaning just barely. "That makes my hide crawl," we say, indicating revulsion or fear. "No sweat!" we say, meaning there's nothing to worry about. "Don't get in a lather!" we caution, meaning there's nothing to get excited about. "He got pale as a ghost" or "red as a beet," we remark. We even realize, perhaps somewhat dimly, that a pimple or a cold sore may herald some internal disorder, usually transient in nature—a stomach upset, we tell ourselves, or a cold coming on. More tragically, sometimes our skin prophesies diseases far more serious, such as cancer.

Thus, we do pay attention to the signals our inner selves project via the skin. Our skin is the barrier, the battlements that stand between ourselves and our world. It is also our jailhouse wall that keeps us imprisoned. Some of us may cower behind our skin like frightened, cornered animals. And some of us may preen ourselves through our skin, painting it brightly, smoothing it, scenting it, loving our hide even as we love ourselves. Some of us, though, turn on our skin savagely, picking at it, rubbing it raw, tearing at it as though to get at our inner selves, which we appear to despise. And then, all of us receive our first and perhaps our last great sense of love and compassion through our skin.

Whatever happens to our skin can be vitally important to all the rest of us. Conversely, what is important to all the rest of us may be mirrored by our skin—our emotions and our allergy, for instance.

As far as we know, the dog scratching by the curb is not suffering emotional overlay to his skin problem, be it flea bites or eczema. Nor, do we think, does the cow who sports hives have some psychological problem. These would seem to be clearly allergic reactions, the skin manifesting the symptoms of an antibody-allergen clash. But when it comes to humans, the picture is never so clear.

To begin with, the skin is much more complex than it looks. It contains among other things sweat glands, nerves, nerve endings, blood vessels, all of which can be affected by emotional stress. The sweat glands, for example, may respond to the physical stimuli of heat or exertion, or to the stimuli of emotions such as anxiety or anger. In movies our hero's face is always bathed profusely in sweat to help portray moments of great danger and/or of physical exertion, and/or of pain from an injury suffered in the course of his heroic action.

Why do such strong emotions as fear, anger, pain, and tension stimulate the sweating response? They do so because the sweat glands are regulated by the sympathetic nervous system, which responds, as we have seen, to impulses sent out by the hypothalamus, which responds in turn to our higher intellect when it recognizes good cause for these emotions. The hypothalamus monitors body temperature, which in turn is regulated by the body's cooling system, the sweat glands. Strong emotions appear to signal for sweat-gland activity in the same manner. Such a response is quite normal and only becomes abnormal when it gets out of hand, so to speak. An example of such abnormality would be excessive sweating or sweating in unusual areas of the body, profuse sweating of the feet, for instance.

In much the same manner, the blood vessels of the skin respond to such strong emotions. We are all familiar with the phenomenon of blushing. Commonly we associate it with the emotion of embarrassment and assume a certain naiveté or guilt on the part of the blusher. It is possible nobody does much blushing anymore. However, we can turn a lovely shade of red or pink equally well by eating spicy tacos or by taking a hot bath or by imbibing one-too-many cocktails. I often have patients, children or women mainly, who when they become nervous turn a speckled sort of red, especially over the chest and shoulders. Generally, we distinguish a flush from a blush—the former being a sudden overall feeling of warmth such as women feel during the hot flashes of menopause, whereas the latter is usually confined to the face, neck, and upper chest. Both, however, are the result of the dilation of blood vessels in the skin, and both can occur among any of us. Blushing and flushing are abnormal symptoms only when they occur too frequently (a difficult criterion to determine) or as an adjunct of disease, such as a flush of fever.

Blanching or turning pale is an opposing phenomenon occurring when the blood vessels of the skin constrict. Again this is an entirely normal response to the stimuli of cold or shock or fear or my skin tests with a fearsome needle.

All in all, our skin mirrors our emotions rather well—and in two-tone color at that. There is nothing out of the ordinary in this. It was made to be so. The other side of the coin, however, is that the condition of our skin can greatly influence our emotional health, perhaps simply because it is the outer wrapping with which we present ourselves to the world. No one wishes to appear repulsive or ugly; thus, it is no easy thing to be even temporarily disfigured by wheals and bumps and rashes. Weeping, pus-laden, crusting lesions are not socially acceptable, while scratching in public like an old hound dog is generally frowned upon. Our self-image is pretty important to our emotional stability, and it is difficult to be debonair and self-confident when the exposed parts of one's body—face, hands, neck, and the like—are sporting lesions or rashes or both. Disorders of the skin are apt to be double-barreled, combining itching and pain with unsightliness. In fact, the itch of eczema and of hives, the inflammation and rawness of contact dermatitis can change our personality by robbing us of sleep and of our sense of general wellbeing. Altogether, disorders of the skin are no subject for amusement. Some individuals have been known to consider suicide because of protracted and severe skin problems, while some skin conditions have been so painful and so intractable as to lead to outright mental illness.

This last urges me to digress a bit to one aspect of the relationship of our emotions to our skin, and it is admittedly a strange and bizarre connection. Many mentally ill patients and mentally deficient persons inflict self-mutilation on their skin as if driven by impulses of self-destruction. They dig and pick and rub and gnaw at their skin, creating such unsightly wounds and growths as "gnaw warts" (horny growths caused by constant chewing at one spot) on their fingers, or patches of thick hair on arms and even on occasion legs where they constantly bite at one small area, or open sores that refuse to heal because of endless picking and the like. The results can be pretty horrendous for the observer and a great trial for the physician in charge of such individuals.

Before we leave the cause of skin manifestations to pass on to the emotional-trigger concept in skin allergies, we should perhaps note the strange mystery of the stigmata, the wounds of Christ that appear for as yet no known organic reason in some deeply religious people. One of the most famous recent cases of such stigmatization is that of Theresa Neumann of Germany. Born on Good Friday, she began to develop the wounds of Christ every Good Friday from the age of twenty-eight on. She was studied assiduously by a host of medical men, but no satisfactory explanation for her stigmata has yet been offered.

However, we do have a somewhat analogous phenomenon in the anniversary syndrome or "special day blues." On these occasions, perhaps because they mark the death of someone dearly loved or of some other sad event, or even perhaps because they denote the day of a happy event since gone sour, some individuals undergo special and often intense emotional stress, so intense sometimes as to trigger symptoms of illness, physical as well as mental, allergy as well as other illnesses.

Well, on to the role of emotions in skin *allergy*. I believe this role is significant and in some cases a strong and compelling factor. There are three main allergic skin conditions that we will discuss here—eczema, urticaria (hives), and contact dermatitis. We will arbitrarily place angiodema (giant hives) in the urticaria slot since it really is a more severe form of the same manifestation. Some allergists insist that emotions play their greatest role in eczema, others are equally insistent that they influence urticaria most, and there are some who believe emotional disturbance is behind almost every skin disorder. I myself tread carefully when it comes to asserting single or prime causes. There is always the story of the patient who scratched like fury, claiming with undiminished stubbornness that there were bugs on his skin. Not a bug was visible, but when the patient reported that he exercised regularly in a room with a window air vent opening on a chickenyard, the doctor in charge took a magnifying glass to the problem. Yep! Chicken mites, sucked into the room by the air vent. Such things make believers out of doctors!

Oddly enough, going through the procedure of taking skin scrapings and observing them under the microscope can be very reassuring for the patient who believes himself infested by bugs of one kind or another, even if they are in reality a figment of his suggestible imagination. It is not only that he may be reassured that everything is being done for him that can be, every avenue explored, so to speak; but in our age of technology the use of scientific instruments wields great powers of infallibility. We moderns are more inclined to put our trust in the wisdom of the machine than in our own brand of intelligence. I have had such patients for whom it is not enough to say that there *are no* bugs. So I have them bring me a piece of skin (or even fluff or dust) in an envelope to prove their contention that bugs are eating them alive. Alas, even when they peer into the microscope themselves, they are sometimes pretty hard to convince that they are bugless.

It may really seem to victims of eczema that *something* is literally eating them alive! The itching can be fierce, so much so that the victim may scratch himself bloody. In fact, some allergists believe that the lesions of eczema are the result not so much of the condition itself as of the patient's digging and scratching to get at the itch. As a matter of fact, the itch alone may be the first and only symptom and thus may represent a puzzle until a rash appears. Eczema also often begins simply as a patch of itching skin followed by a slight reddening of the area, and then the whole thing may begin to spread in an exceedingly disconcerting manner. In infants, eczema most often makes its appearance on the face, usually on the cheeks or around the ears. In older children and adults it may show up initially on the inner arms or the back of the knees, then go on to involve the face, neck, chest, scalp, and the backs of the hands. In time the patches of reddish rash may turn brown and thicken. In chronic cases, such skin changes may never completely disappear. In all of this, that intense itching we spoke of drives the eczema sufferer to excesses of scratching. This often causes extensive abrasions accompanied by weeping and crusting, with secondary infection a likely result. Severe eczema can make a mess of one's hide and, as we noted earlier, rob one of sleep, jangle one's nerves, and be a source of embarrassment and depression. If the patient was emotionally disturbed before the appearance of his eczema, he is sure to be doubly so after it surfaces!

As with asthma, all that itches is not eczema and all that is eczema is not necessarily allergic in origin. Technically, what we are concerned with here is atopic dermatitis, eczema resulting from sensitivity to an allergen. However, if we all understand that this is what we are discussing, then let us call it simply eczema and make less of a mouthful for ourselves. Eczema has a habit of making its debut in childhood, often during the first six months of life. Frequently it will spontaneously disappear when the child is around three only to pop out again as the child nears puberty. It is believed that from 1 to 3 percent of children under age two suffer from eczema and that one-half to three quarters of these sufferers have a family history of allergy. Unhappily, somewhere around 50 percent of the youngsters who suffer early eczema go on to hay fever and/or asthma. This is why we consider eczema the leader in the "allergic march," the progression from eczema to colic to asthma which often appears among allergic children. It is quite usual to find the older eczema patient also troubled by other allergies, especially allergy of the respiratory system.

Eczema, then, should be taken seriously apart from its own general discomfort and possible emotional trauma. In one long-term, follow-up study of 40 individuals who suffered eczema in childhood, 14 still suffered from it 20 years later, 11 had gone on to develop asthma, while 18 had moved to hay fever. Worse still, half of the group had moved to a stage in which they suffered chronically from all three allergies—a full complement of curses! Out of the 40 only 11 went on to adulthood scot-free and to stay that way for the 20-year period of the study. That's not a very good track record for early eczema.

Probably most infantile eczema begins as allergy to cow's milk, and much of it can be controlled simply by changing the baby's formula or by using heat-treated milk (evaporated, for instance), which is far less allergenic. Eggs and wheat may start up the itch-scratch syndrome a little later when they are introduced into the youngster's diet. The children who react in this fashion will also commonly be sensitive to inhalants and sometimes to drugs. What, if any, role the emotions play in infantile eczema is questionable. At this stage, the largest controlling factor other than allergens is probably the presence of an infection. Sometimes when an eczematous child loses his infected tonsils or adenoids, he also loses his eczema.

When we follow eczema into later childhood, adolescence especially, and into adulthood, the factors involved take on a different aspect. The primary cause remains an allergen or allergens, usually foods or inhalants, but emotional stress may aggravate the condition considerably. First, let's examine the itch itself. What in the world is it?

Ogden Nash wrote one of his inimitable limericks about the young belle of Natchez whose clothes become patches because when she itches she scratches. (See his "Requiem.") The Chinese invented a special tool to get at an itch in the middle of the back, a spot where only backing up to a door jamb can be effective without this wonder of eastern invention. Anyone who has suffered through a bout of summertime agony in the form of poison ivy is able to sympathize with the eczema victim. But the itch itself is strange. If you put your mind hard to it, it's difficult to explain in words just what it is. It is not pain. It is even pleasure to scratch at it, yet often pain will follow on the heels of that pleasure. Technically, the skin registers only four fundamental sensations–pain, touch, heat, and cold. So, actually, it is believed that an itch is pain, or at least so closely related that we can say it *is* pain of a very low intensity. Studies of people who have lost their sense of pain indicate that they have also lost their ability to itch, which seems an odd trade-off. It is what actually causes this low level of pain that stumps the researchers. Most seem to lean to the theory that chemical substances are released which set up a series of electrical impulses in the skin and that brings the sensation of itching. We do know that in allergic eczema in the skin area affected there is a rise in the level of such mediators as histamine, whereas in the skin areas unaffected by eczema, the level appears to remain normal. What we don't know about eczema and its itching, however, greatly outweighs what we can say with any certainty, so perhaps we should paraphrase Gertrude Stein: an itch is an itch is an itch.

As for scratching, we don't even know why it temporarily relieves the itch, but it does. However, we do know that too-vigorous scratching can make the itch worse by bringing about an increase in the chemicals that probably triggered the itch in the first place. So–whether scratching interrupts nerve messages of itching to the brain or momentarily substitutes a higher level of pain sensation for the low level of itching–whatever you do, if you *must* scratch, scratch gently. In fact, don't scratch, stroke! Stroke with the palm of your hand and leave your fingernails out of it. You might also try rubbing the area around the itch, rather than on the itching spot itself. This often will bring not only the same measure of relief, but the relief will last longer. (See Appendix F for a list of do's and don't's in this matter)

There are some oddities about eczema's mighty itch. One recent study demonstrated that eczema patients go right on scratching in their sleep. The investigators even measured the intervals of such scratching and came up with the figure that some 4 percent of sleep time is devoted to this activity. That's a lot of nighttime scratching! Even more interesting is the finding that such scratching occurred even in the period of deepest sleep when emotional stress would be minimal. Conversely, it did not occur during the "rapid eye movement" level of sleep when emotional content appears to be at its highest. This would seem to confirm the physical primary cause of atopic dermatitis, or our brand of eczema as it were.

It has been suggested that the eczematous patient possesses a fundamentally more irritable or unstable skin than normal (just as it has been suggested that the asthma patient possesses more irritable or unstable bronchi than the nonasthmatic individual). Thus, the victim of eczema would register the impact of various stimuli more intensely. He would also, it is suggested, become more easily habituated or conditioned to the itch-scratch syndrome, although this is still open to considerable question.

I want to note here an interesting comment by a colleague who administers an alcohol treatment unit. He has noticed that some of his patients who are suffering from exceedingly severe eczema when they begin treatment improve markedly after they cut out alcohol. It is possible, my colleague remarks, that this phenomenon could be due to improved nutrition. Whatever the reason, it's an interesting proposition, especially since many allergists interested in the role of foods in allergic diseases have pointed a finger at the ingredients of beer, wine, and hard liquor as being reasonably potent allergens. There has even been the suggestion that some alcoholics are essentially allergic, and that their alcoholism may even be a symptom of allergy disease. However, this hypothesis is by no means certain as yet. We have still a lot to learn about both conditions.

Well, is eczema a psychosomatic illness? One school of thought suggests that the psychosomatic factor is very large indeed. Studies are cited that indicate very disturbed child-parent relationships among many young eczema sufferers and various personality disorders among adult eczema patients. Proponents of the psychosomatic theory in eczema suggest that the itch-scratch syndrome is an abnormal adaption to chronic anxiety, that it is a form of regressive behavior in the teeth of unresolved conflict and latent hostility.

Personally I don't believe the psychosomatic view of eczema is totally valid. While emotional stress obviously plays a large role, I believe it is clearly secondary to that of allergens. Scratching within limits does seem to be a normal response to mental and emotional stimuli. We scratch our heads when thinking through some puzzle or idea. We may scratch the back of our hands or an ear when pondering a decision. We sometimes scratch our noses when excited, simply because they may itch during such moments. Since eczematous individuals go on to scratch themselves raw, such abnormality may be a matter of degree, an allergic condition aggravated by emotional stress.

Nor do I believe that there is a clear-cut eczema personality so that we can say, when confronted by such a person, "Aha, this fellow will develop eczema! This is an eczematous person!" However, I do agree that an eczematous person is vulnerable to emotional stress, that his underlying predisposition can be triggered by the emotions most often attributed to eczema—frustration and repressed hostility. For example, in one study in which eczematous patients were asked a number of questions and the results compared to similar questionnaires given a control group of dental patients with no prior history of eczema, the eczematous patients revealed more stressful life events in their recent pasts than the dental patients. It also indicated that more of them were disturbed to a much greater extent by such events than the dental patients and that psychologically they might have been more vulnerable to such emotional disturbances because of early childhood separation from a parent. Interestingly enough, the eczematous patients also admitted to being angry and frustrated more often than members of the control group. All of these, of course, were subjective findings in the main.

One theory that I find rather fascinating is the proposition that the eczema sufferer may be predisposed to his affliction because his mother did not hold and snuggle him enough in infancy. How one goes about "proving" such a theory is difficult to say. Perhaps a study of different cultures would illustrate that eczema might turn up to a much lesser degree among, say, people who habitually carry their babies in slings against their bodies or the like.

Proponents of the personality-profile theory can even tell you what the eczematous victim will look like. Frequently, they say, he will be tall and lean, not very muscular, and he will sweat very little. They go on to say that he will be nervous, restless, more intelligent than average, and that he will lack self-confidence and be dependent and insecure.

If we go back to examine the other side of the coin, which we touched on briefly earlier in the chapter, we may find that the eczema sufferer has good reason for some of his manifestations of emotional distress. People who are somewhat susceptible to mosquito bites will have good insight into the tortures of a severe and constant itch. And when the face or hands become unsightly under the digging and scratching, when the lesions weep and crust, then we can surely understand that the eczema patient is going to be embarrassed, his sense of self-esteem and self-confidence diminished. It is not difficult to imagine what even temporary disfigurement can do to one's self-image, and eczema can be pretty horrendous on occasion. The sufferer may even feel dirty or repulsive to others at times. Add to this the irritability from loss of sleep and constant itching and you have a pretty thoroughly stressed patient. If his eczema is chronic and prolonged, he may withdraw from social contacts and become subdued and depressed. He may doubt his own sanity when he reads or hears about self-destructive impulses, or when people infer that he is taking out his repressed hostility on himself.

There is another factor here that should be mentioned. The eczema patient may also be suffering from other allergies (which won't help his emotional set any). For instance, I am treating a ten-year-old boy for several allergies. His mother says that whenever he gets upset or mad, he begins to scratch and his eczema flares up. While his anger may trigger eczema, the prime cause is his allergic condition already manifested in other allergy symptoms. I have warned his mother to be careful not to let him use his eczema to get his way, just as the asthma patient does on occasion. We will go on to discuss the importance of child-parent relationships in allergy in a later chapter. We will also try to find an answer for the question posed in the following letter from a very perceptive eczema sufferer:*

> I am a long time sufferer of atopic dermatitis. I find it is adversely affected by high summer humidity in New Jersey, and by my choice of whether or not to experience and express rage and anger. If I choose in the moment of irritation to experience anger I seldom have symptoms. Or [I] can

*Frederick Gardner, Media Decisions, 342 Madison Avenue, New York, N.Y. 10017.

> consciously repress and have the anger expressed by expanding capillaries and subsequent itching, drying and peeling. . . . There are times when I *would* rather itch than be angry. The question is how do I and others with allergies program themselves for more constructive forms of self-expression that are compatible with our personalities and life styles?

Let's hold the phone and tackle this question later, for it is relevant not only to eczema but to all allergies in which emotions play a significant role. In fact, it is relevant to a good many other diseases as well.

When we come to urticaria, the slightly melodic medical term for hives, we may find first the wheals and then the itch, or we may first feel the itch and then find the wheals, which are pale bumps often circled in red that pop out suddenly on the skin. The name of this quite common skin disorder comes from the Latin word meaning nettle. If you have ever waded through a stand of nettles barelegged, you will have an excellent feel for an attack of hives! But, again, all that wheals is not allergy. Hives may be caused by parasitic infestation or may signal more serious illnesses such as tumors.

One brand of hives called cholinergic urticaria is not, as far as we know at present, a manifestation of allergy. It seems to arise from physical alterations caused by sheer emotional disturbance. So do hives that pop out when the hypersensitive person is exposed to sudden drops in temperature or after exertion. It is not necessarily severe cold, interestingly enough, that produces hives in such people, but their extreme sensitivity to a sudden drop in temperature. Even drinking a glass of cold water can bring the wheals popping out!

Hives appear on various parts of the body but most frequently on flat surfaces such as the chest, back, the planes of forearms and legs. They may cover only a small area or be extensive. In an acute attack of hives new ones may keep appearing as the old fade away. In chronic cases, they come, stick around for a few hours or days, then vanish. They are often accompanied by angioedema, a more deep-seated swelling. This odd condition can transform a charming face into a grotesque mask or be so generalized as to increase body size. One doctor reports a woman patient subject to this overall reaction who had to keep three sets of clothing of varying sizes handy to accomodate her changing measurements. Angioedema was once widely known as angioneurotic edema because of its apparent correlation with emotional disturbance, but probably most allergists today believe allergy accounts for a majority of cases. We should note that angioedema of the larynx area can be exceedingly dangerous. It can cause death by suffocation. Fortunately, such involvement is relatively rare.

So what part do emotions play in urticaria and angioedema? In truth, research into this question has not been extensive to date, although I think most allergists would agree that emotional stress plays a large role indeed. Some feel that it is possible that psychogenic factors may be the prime cause for both skin disorders, that most cases of hives are cholinergic. In any case, we do know that patients often develop urticaria at the time of or just after some stress condition and that hives may well persist after all possible allergenic substances have cleared the individual's system. We also know that in the production of hives, organic changes in the skin occur: the blood vessels dilate, leaking fluid into the tissues with an accompanying rise in skin temperature. When such changes occur suddenly, an allergic reaction is usually at the bottom of the trouble, but when urticaria is chronic, things become uncertain. Even here, in the majority of cases, I believe, an allergen could be found at work; but as we noted, there is a type of urticaria that may be purely emotional in origin. For example, in one study of 40 chronic urticaria sufferers, no allergens or other physical cause for their distress could be found. The researchers also demonstrated that most, if not all, of these patients suffered from emotional stress, anxiety in particular. It was concluded that these individuals had resorted, not consciously, of course, to a conversion of their fears to the physical symptoms of hives. I suppose the itch-scratch cycle would be bound to take at least a part of your mind from your troubles. Even more possible is the fact that some people with sensitive skin can raise a good crop of hives by just rubbing or scratching. There is even a condition called dermographia in which elongated wheals can be raised on the skin simply by stroking it with a tongue depressor or other blunt instrument. One can even write one's name on the back of a patient whose skin can register such sensitivity. Whether or not this is an allergic reaction is not really known with any certainty. If it is, it would come under the heading of physical allergy—hypersensitivity to friction as well as to heat and cold and light. A certain amount of controversy still rages around the allergic basis for physical allergy, in any case.

What emotions play a role in skin allergy in particular? As in asthma, suppressed weeping has been ascribed to urticaria. Like the asthmatic individual, the urticaria patient is considered to be dependent, anxious about the loss of the maternal figure or about being abandoned, and frustrated. Certainly, as we have noted, there are individuals who possess skin so sensitive that they register not only physical stimuli but also the stimulus of emotional stress with its actual physical alterations. And since once the itch-scratch cycle begins, it tends to perpetuate itself, individuals who are inclined to repress their feelings and turn inward may also be likely to turn against themselves and manipulate or abuse their skin to produce a crop of hives. Certain emotional stresses do give rise to self-destructive impulses.

Since skin temperature rises in urticaria, one study made use of this fact to test a group of 20 hypnotized subjects who were not inclined to develop hives to determine if *their* skin temperature could be raised. It was suggested to them (under hypnosis) that they were being mistreated and were helpless to alter the situation. This, it was thought, would replicate the typical anxiety and frustration often seen in the chronic urticaria patient. These suggestions, carried out on two separate days, did raise skin temperatures significantly. When these same patients were told that they desired to strike out at someone or something (an emotion considered to aggrevate hypertension, by the way), their skin temperatures fell. This study demonstrated two differing physical reactions in the skin to two quite different emotional inputs; or, at any rate, in individuals under the influence of hypnosis.

Well, we are back to the old question of whether emotions can "cause" hives or are simply a "trigger." I suppose I must commit myself. We do know that we can produce hives by injecting histamine under the skin, and thus duplicate in a way the allergic mechanism. We also know that the central nervous system can dictate the release of such histamine into the skin (in a somewhat roundabout way), so that this mechanism can be initiated by the physical responses to emotional stress. Therefore, I believe that while the majority of urticaria patients are truly allergic, some may suffer from hives for psychogenic reasons. I also believe that frequently it is a matter of the two factors acting together, especially in the case of chronic urticaria. As in eczema, the possibility that the mechanism becomes habituated or conditioned seems great.

So, is there a urticaria personality? Proponents say, yes, there is. He is a somewhat passive fellow given to strong masochistic tendencies. He takes powerful feelings of resentment and frustration out on his own hide. Like the asthmatic individual he has difficulty weeping, but when he does weep, his urticaria symptoms diminish or are terminated–sometimes suddenly with the onset of tears! He would appear to be Dr. Bell's avoider or perhaps the pleaser, both of whom suffer much at their own hands, it seems.

Before we leave urticaria, and just as a matter of interest, it can be mentioned that hives occur much more frequently in women than in men; they infrequently appear before the age of ten, but most often seem to arrive in the period from the twenties to the beginning of old age. They are relatively rare in senior citizens. What we are to make of these facts I'm not sure.

In a culture where contact with chemical and metal substances is bountiful, we not surprisingly have an exceedingly high incidence of contact dermatitis, skin conditions brought on by sensitivity to various environmental factors. The natural world produces its own brand of booby trap also, poison ivy being probably the best known. Some people are so sensitive to these three shiny leaves which grace the American landscape so plentifully that hospitalization may be required. Many people suffer more moderately, while a few people can actually pick it and take home a bouquet without so much as an itch. Once sensitized, however, the individual will probably retain his allergic reaction for many years, even for his lifetime.

Contact dermatitis turns up in the middle-aged and elderly more frequently than in the young, perhaps because of more frequent exposure to a variety of substances. It does not seem to run in families as a tendency as do other allergies. Nor does it seem to have a close connection to emotional stress. What emotional disturbance accompanies its symptoms seems in most cases to arise from the symptoms themselves. For instance, contact dermatitis in older people can be a cause for a good bit of anxiety. They may interpret it as a life threat and as a sign of more serious illness. Thus, elderly patients are apt to be fearful and uncooperative with the doctor. Also it is generally more difficult to treat among older people and has a habit of lingering for some good time. Thus, older contact dermatitis patients are apt to get pretty depressed before the skin is cleared. Not only that, but many tend to be suspicious of the shaman's skill and stubborn about the nature of their problem, insisting that something is causing it which is not at all germane to their condition. Such notions make the problem of avoidance of the irritating substance an iffy business, and the wise shaman may have to employ the same sort of psychology he would need for a recalcitrant mule. If you want to go in one certain direction, you head the mule on an opposing compass point! The fact that such elderly patients may have been in contact with the substance for years doesn't help matters. The suddenness of their symptoms only increases their doubt in the doctor's intelligence.

For example, I treated a woman who was well into her eighties in spite of her jet black hair. She was suffering considerable dermatitis of the face, particularly around the hair line. I inquired tactfully if she used hair dye. "Oh, no, never! How can you even suggest such a thing!" However, a bit of testing told a different story and she finally confessed. As her hair resumed its normal color, so the skin of her face returned to its very pleasant texture. We wise shamans need tact and patience and the ability to deliver a good simple lecture on the phenomenon of sensitization.

Another woman patient arrived with dermatitis of the eyelids and bright red fingernails. "Aha," I said to her, "You're allergic to your fingernail polish." "Impossible!" she cried, glancing at me askance. "How would I get polish on my eyelids?" "Rubbing them," I replied in my inimitable Sherlock manner. "Well, why isn't this rash all over my fingers?" "Because the skin of your eyelids is much thinner and more sensitive. Better try a different brand or, better still, no polish at all." However, when it comes to cosmetics, women are hard to convince.

It is not difficult to understand that contact dermatitis, particularly when it affects the face, neck, and hands, can trail some potent emotional stresses in its wake, even as can eczema and urticaria. When we are "blemished" by whatever cause, minor emotional problems are likely to become major, as our self-image is distorted and diminished, our self-confidence shattered. Social anxieties are very real and often harsh. If we trip carrying coffee to the pastor in the parlor and dump a cupful in his lap, we may be intensely and momentarily embarrassed, but later we will probably find much to laugh about in the incident. But when we present to our peers encrusted, scabbing cheeks or hands sloughing patches of hide, our emotional stress (and their dismay) can be excruciating. There does not appear to be any appropriate apology for our condition or any room for future amusement. To wear a mask or hide behind a newspaper or the like is only apt to make matters worse by calling even more attention to our plight. I once treated a young girl with long-standing eczema of the hands. The poor youngster wore white gloves from morning to night—to school, to meals, in the gym. Quite naturally, everyone she met wanted to know why. Since her anguish was considerable, if I had not been able to clear up her eczema with reasonable dispatch, she might conceivably have become mentally ill. It is by no means rare for a patient suffering from such exposed skin involvement to sink into a severe depression, even to such an extent as to consider suicide. Most of us are well aware of the emotional trauma acne (not an allergic condition, incidentally) can inflict on the adolescent and how it can even color the future personality of the adult. Young people and/or their parents spend millions of dollars annually in search of acne's good riddance!

Back in Chapter 3 I described two ladies, Judith P., who suffered contact dermatitis caused by a harsh detergent, and Jane T., who suffered from chronic eczema. You will remember that while Judith was upset by the state of her hands, her emotional stress, such as it was, vanished with her dermatitis. Jane, on the other hand, although clearly allergic, had so many built-in emotional problems that even medication and control measures were unlikely to clear up her symptoms permanently. To understand why this might be so, let us say that Jane's eczema began in infancy and has continued on a chronic basis ever since. Somewhere in the course of these many years, Jane has met some harsh realities, beginning perhaps with her mother's revulsion before her child's messy skin. Such a rejection would brand its scar for a lifetime. Add to it the probable reaction of Jane's peers to her eczema, and you will be able to imagine the powerful emotional distress such revulsion and rejection could create, the unhappiness, the diminished self-esteem and self-confidence, the probable withdrawal from contact with others, the dependency even in adult years upon the mother, the turning in on oneself. Denied other pleasures, Jane may have found at least some pleasure in scratching, and/or it may have become a mechanism to hit out at her own body to relieve frustration and anger at a cruel, rejecting world, and/or it may have served to distract her attention from the anguish of her problem. Eczema became a way of life, and as such it will persist.

I think, then, we can say that Jane's eczema, begun as an allergic response to allergenic substances, became chronic under the pressures of emotional stress. Many allergists have noted that allergic symptoms that arise in childhood and persist into adulthood often show a significant correlation with various life crises, crises such as puberty, leaving home for college or the service or an occupation, marriage, menopause, the loss of someone dear, and the like. For some reason as yet unclear, it seems possible that emotional stimuli may take the place of the allergens that were originally responsible for the allergic response or symptoms. To be frank about it, no one is certain, for there are a variety of other factors that may enter here—our biological rhythms, for instance, infection, genetic predisposition, and so on. The matter is complex and there are no single answers.

In any case, the reader must be fully aware by now of the importance of treating the allergic patient as a whole, that he is not an isolated itch, or lesion, or desire to scratch. He is a complex combination of these characteristics and much, much more.

12
Gastrointestinal Allergy and Emotional Upset

"Oh dear," she cried, "that man made me so angry I have butterflies in my stomach!"

"What he said sure sticks in my craw!" he agreed. "I just can't stomach that man!"

"Every time he opens his mouth, he makes my gorge rise!" she concurred, frowning. "But let's forget about *him,* darling. Let's go have that marvelous dinner at the Beau Ritz that you promised me. Candlelight and soft music. The works."

So off they went, and as the reader may have already guessed, their evening out wasn't going to be all that enjoyable in the long run. Oh, the menu was a marvel, the linen soft and white as snow, the candle mellow, the music romantic, the cuisine superb, the service quietly elegant, the check astronomical. Pleasure was theirs, for a while, but pain followed on its heels a few hours later.

"It must have been the onions in cream sauce," she announced the next morning over a skimpy (by choice) breakfast. "First, I felt nauseated and then everything just churned and churned. The whole night through. Or at least it felt like it. I should have known better. I never have any luck with onions, and that cream sauce was much too rich!"

"Gosh," he exclaimed, surprised, "I thought I was the only one in trouble! I thought it was the shrimp with me. Maybe they weren't . . . . Oh, no, that's not possible at that price!"

This duet could go on and on. I want to add hastily that in truth the shrimp were marvelously fresh and the onions couldn't have been more delicious. It wasn't the fault of the chef or the restaurant. No dread botulism or unpleasant salmonella lurked in their meal. Many other diners ate heartily of shrimp and creamed onions that evening and slept the whole night through. Of course, she may have had an intolerance to onions as some people do (and to beans and prunes and spinach and the like), but what really caused their pleasure to turn to pain was allergy—hers to milk (in the *creamed* onions) and his to shellfish. Both their allergies were mild and ordinarily they might have developed no symptoms, but unfortunately they took their anger and resentment to dinner with them. Not surprisingly, considering what we have learned from peeking into Tom's stomach "window," this emotional disturbance altered their digestive processes. Even if they had not been allergic, they might have had repercussions from such rich fare devoured during a time of emotional stress. On the other hand, they might have had nothing but pleasure from their meal if they had expressed their anger or physically attacked the source, the gentleman in question. It is the suppressed rage that can cause inflammation of the gastrointestinal tract. This, in turn, seems to allow greater penetration of food allergens into the mucous membranes and blood vessels. In the case of our dining couple, this meant a breaching of their allergic threshold and gastrointestinal allergy symptoms.

As far as we can determine the antibody-allergen struggle takes place directly in the gastrointestinal tract, when a number of things appear to happen to the tissues of whatever section of the GI tract has been sensitized previously by the allergen in question. In one study, allergic patients examined with a gastroscope (a tool to examine one's innards) after ingesting an allergenic food exhibited inflammation and swelling of the gastrointestinal mucosa. Nodes or aggregates of cells appeared, along with a thickening of mucous membrane folds. Peristalsis, that wavelike motion of the gastrointestinal tract that shunts our nourishment along like a switch engine on a freight yard, diminished, and there was a great outpouring of mucous secretions. All of this normally happened within two hours of ingestion of the allergenic food. It should be noted that in this study of what happens to the GI tract of such patients, the allergenic food was disguised to rule out any possibility of suggestion.

The gastrointestinal tract can sport allergy symptoms from mouth to anus. Sometimes only one part of the system is affected, but more commonly several areas are involved. Symptoms can be exceedingly severe or they can be so mild and diffuse as to generate simply a generalized sense of unwellness and discomfort. Some allergists believe gastrointestinal allergic reactions are rather rare; others think they are far more common than generally acknowledged. Since such a reaction is a less well known manifestation of allergy than asthma or hay fever, eczema or hives, perhaps we should present a brief rundown of symptoms.

Starting with the mouth in a natural progression of parts, we note that an allergic reaction can result in an itching, burning sensation in the mouth with swelling of lips, tongue, gums, and pharynx. (We noted earlier in our discussion of angioedema that this last symptom of allergy can be life threatening when severe.) The skin around the mouth may break out in dermatitis, and the lips be chapped or inflamed. One odd symptom that could turn up is "geographical" tongue, so called because the patchy appearance of the tongue somewhat resembles a map. Often the above symptoms are accompanied by a bad taste in the mouth and, unhappily, that bugaboo of social encounter, bad breath. Perhaps the most annoying symptom of all is the appearance of canker sores. These lesions in and around the mouth frequently turn up as a sensitivity to some foods, drugs, and on occasion the use of tobacco. If more smokers had this particular problem, they might live longer! Unhappily, some of the flavorings used in mouthwashes and toothpaste can also produce these sores in sensitive individuals, and some unfortunates can react to their dentures in this fashion.

As far as I know there has been little if any study of the role of emotions in producing such symptoms about the mouth area, but the reader can imagine how such swellings and lesions, bad taste, and bad breath can trail emotional stress in their wake. We are pursued by commercial advertising that equates bad breath with social sin, and we are repeatedly admonished to disguise our facial imperfections, temporary or permanent, beneath a layer of goo. Some of this rather naturally rubs off on our ideas of social acceptance, so that we find our self-image diminished when such imperfections appear. Few of us are debonair enough to meet the world calmly with grossly swollen lips or a tongue that looks like the map of Europe.

When the antibody-allergen struggle takes place in the throat area, it can produce symptoms of difficulty in swallowing, a sensation of suddenly possessing a lump under the breast bone which can sometimes be painful, an urge to constantly clear the throat, and coughing due to an increase in mucous secretions. These last two are not necessarily nervous manifestations, although it has to be admitted that once started, throat clearing and coughing can become habitual and be stimulated by nervousness. All of these symptoms are somewhat nebulous and are all too often dismissed as hypochondria, especially when there are no other accompanying symptoms of allergy. In fact, so much of a mild gastrointestinal allergic reaction is so diffuse and obscure that the patient's complaints, if he bothers to voice any, often sound like those of a veteran hypochondriac.

Nausea, vomiting, heartburn, sour sensations, bloating, belching—all may indicate an allergic reaction in the stomach area. Certainly they are all familiar symptoms; if we haven't experienced them firsthand, we find them hourly on the TV screen in commercials that vividly present belching bottles and beakers and the agonized faces of actors going through the motions of internal misery. Such picturesque seething and stewing can be the result of dietary indiscretion, but it can also indicate an allergy to foods. Unhappily for the allergic victims, most often the everyday varieties of foods cause the most trouble—milk, eggs, wheat, and corn.

As we have noted, we also know (thanks to Tom's window) that changes occur in the mucus of the stomach and intestinal tract under the whipsaw of powerful emotions. And, as we have noted, such alterations appear to make the stomach and intestinal mucus more vulnerable to allergenic substances. Thus, to try to separate prime cause and contributing factor for all this seething and stewing is a difficult task. It gets no simpler as we contemplate intestinal symptoms sometimes so painful that they mimic appendicitis or obstruction. Such allergic sufferers have been wheeled into surgery on occasion for operations to correct these conditions, only to find that surgery wasn't required. Abdominal pain, diarrhea, constipation, mucus, and even blood in the stool may all be a result of either emotional stress or allergic reaction.

Is this confusing? Mystifying? If the answer is yes, and I expect that it is, I shall be truthful and admit a trade secret—a good many of us in medicine are equally confused. It is no sin to be flummoxed on occasion. Being entirely human, we doctors love to be able to say firmly and wisely to our patients, "Sir (or Madam), your problem is caused by such and such a virus, bacterium, injury, toxic substance, allergen, and the like. If you will but take this pill, shot, syrup, operation, and the like, you will be well again."

Alas, there are so many occasions, particularly in the field of allergy, when such simplistic approaches do not work. Oh, to be sure, symptoms may vanish temporarily, sometimes just because patients have a habit of looking upon their doctor as a sort of god ordained to make them instantly well. Remissions are not "cures," and we allergists, if we do not have a care, are often bedeviled by relapses. This is especially true if we fail to take all factors into account, mental as well as physical—the whole patient with his entire problem!

However, I am also willing to admit that there are patients—fortunately for my ego and their health, quite rare—for whom even the holistic approach appears useless. I believe that there are some few individuals for whom illness is the only possible adaption to life circumstances, that they cannot lay down their illness without falling into ruin. It becomes a very real question then whether the shaman does them a favor by making them well. And since often enough it is simply not possible for a doctor to change the environment and life style of some of these patients to restore good health, he is bound to fail—which may be just as well, for such a patient, "cured" of one ailment, is sure to move on to another. There simply are people who will cling to illness even if it kills them. Nor do I necessarily mean hypochondria, but rather "real" illness with "real" symptoms, a manipulation in a way, or an organic vulnerability.

The above discussion is somewhat of a digression from gastrointestinal allergy and the role emotions play in its multiple manifestations; yet, since I now propose a second theory, it needed to be said to offset this new proposition: that a far greater number of people suffer from allergy to foods than has generally been recognized. I believe that a good deal of unwellness, both transient and chronic, and a good bit of recurrent impairment of the ability to function emotionally is caused by "hidden" sensitivity to ordinary components of our daily fare. I freely admit that I can't prove this, although I am sure that I could provide a supplemental book twice as thick as this one full of cases of individuals with such sensitivities who have been "restored" to the good life. I think, then, it behooves us to be wary of labeling nebulous symptoms as "poor life adaptions" and the like. Perhaps such illness is a crutch, perhaps not. It's a little like the problem the death penalty poses: can we ever be absolutely sure of a person's guilt? Sometimes, yes, of course. But sometimes maybe not with absolute certainty. So it is, I think, with "hidden" allergy compounded by emotional stress.

Allergy to food is not synonymous with gastrointestinal allergy, for the latter can be caused by drugs and by some inhalants. Food allergens, however, are the prime causes for gastrointestinal allergic symptoms. Sensitivity to them can also be registered on the skin as urticaria and angioedema, in the respiratory system as rhinitis and asthma, or in the central nervous system with a variety of symptoms ranging from headaches to bizarre behavior, as we shall see in the next chapter.

There are two types of allergic reaction to food. The first is a constant and everpresent outbreak of symptoms whenever the offending food is consumed. Usually such symptoms tend to be severe and recur whenever the victim tries to approach such a food allergen. It may be a lifetime sensitivity. Fortunately such reactions are rare.

The most common type of allergic reaction to food is variable, and most likely to be affected by emotional stress and other factors such as infection, weather changes, additional sensitivity to inhalants or drugs, and the like. This is the type suffered by our diners-out who went raging to the dinnertable to eat of the best and suffer the worst! This type of reaction to food may come and go and be affected by the age of its victim, whether the infant hitting his bottle, the youth going through adolescence, the woman passing through menstruation or menopause, the elderly going through the metabolic changes of old age. It is neither necessarily a lifetime proposition nor is it "fixed," occurring predictably whenever a specific amount of the allergenic food is ingested. Rather it is the allergic reaction we pictured on our scales back on pages 65 and 67. It is very likely the source of "hidden" allergy.

Perhaps I have not fully dispelled the reader's wonder that such perfectly good, fresh and wholesome foods as milk, eggs, wheat, and corn can cause gastrointestinal misery, asthma, urticaria, and other symptoms. How can drinking a glass of fresh milk bring on an attack of wheezing? Or eating a slice of nutritious whole wheat bread bring on bloating, belching, and diarrhea? Come on, Dr. Frazier, dogs with hay fever and cows with hives were bad enough!

Well, by way of answer, I will borrow an old maxim attributed to Lucretius, Roman poet and philosopher, who said many centuries ago, "What is food for one, is to others bitter poison." We hear it more often these days as, "One man's meat is another man's poison."

Any food may cause an allergic reaction in someone, but the following are the most potent allergens:

milk	eggs
wheat	corn
shellfish	fish
chocolate	nuts
peas	peanuts
berries	citrus fruits

When individuals have inherited a predisposition to a somewhat inefficient gastrointestinal tract, or when infection or emotional stress transform a normally efficient system into an inefficient and, thus, vulnerable system, sensitization to a food can take place and food allergens can do their dirty work by stirring up the antibodies in the vulnerable area to do battle. In addition, when an individual who possesses a somewhat susceptible gastrointestinal tract consumes large quantities of a potently allergenic food, sensitization may take place. He who eats eggs every morning for breakfast and has a family history of allergy runs more risk than normal. Moderation has special virtue for those with a genetic predisposition to allergy or those whose gastrointestinal tracts may have been made vulnerable by such things as a severe case of measles or an argument with a mother-in-law.

Like other allergies, sensitivity to food can arrive at any time of life, but it turns up most frequently in childhood, especially in infancy, perhaps because such youthful gastrointestinal tracts are pretty inefficient or perhaps because babies and young children consume large quantities of a few foods, i.e., milk and cereals.

Middle age often brings allergic reaction to foods eaten for years. It arrives out of the blue, as it were, which can be puzzling for patient and physician alike. Many a woman passing through menopause who abruptly begins to suffer from obscure symptoms of "indigestion" is told she is simply "nervous" because of hormonal changes. For example, Mrs. X recently was referred to me by her family doctor because of persistent abdominal discomfort–bloating, gas, on-again–off-again diarrhea, and occasional colicky abdominal pain. She had already had extensive GI series tests and the like, and all organic possibilities had been thoroughly explored and ruled out. During this process, several specialists had inferred that her real problem was "all in her head," that she was simply suffering from nerves, a menopausal adjunct as it were. But her family doctor who had known her for years wasn't so sure. He thought, wise man, that there might be a possibility of allergy.

Mrs. X was nervous and upset enough in my office.

"I really don't feel well, Dr. Frazier. I used to feel wonderful. I've always had good health and I never, never had stomach trouble before. Oh, of course, temporary upsets when I let my appetite get out of hand or ate something gone a bit bad." She sighed. "I suppose it's just my nerves and change of life or something, but I hate to not feel well so much of the time . . . ."

"All this began at about the time you entered menopause?" I asked, glancing at her chart.

She nodded. "The odd part is that I really haven't had any trouble otherwise. Nothing like the awful stories you hear. But maybe I am neurotic. I do feel tense and irritable and awfully depressed."

Well, there it was. It could be nerves, the menopause and its attendant emotional imbalances. But it also could be allergy aggravated by the hormonal changes of menopause with emotional disturbances trailed along behind. In any case, it certainly should be explored, so explore we did. We completed a number of lab and skin tests, and while skin testing for food allergy is not reliable, it may nevertheless provide some clues. I also skin-tested for various inhalants on the chance that these, too, could be having a hand in Mrs. X's troubles. I then put Mrs. X on an elimination diet that removed potent allergenic and suspect foods from her daily fare.

Then, having shaken my gourd rattle three times and pronounced a number of magic words, I left the matter pretty much up to Mrs. X for the next few weeks. And that's all it took. Greatly excited, she came in to tell me that her troubles were over, that her "indigestion" had vanished, that she felt great once more. "And," she added happily, "best of all I'm not depressed or even irritable any more. My husband says that I'm my own, sweet self again!"

Aha, I preen a little and take a modest bow. Of course, I am quite aware that things could have turned out differently, that some deep-seated emotional problem could have been at the root of her "indigestion." As it turned out, she was caught up in the allergy–emotional stress–allergy circle, so that what began as mild allergy was aggravated by emotional stress caused by the misinterpretation of and anxiety about her allergic symptoms. On top of all this, hormonal changes were probably lowering her threshold of tolerance to allergens. And this was the case; for we soon discovered, as one by one we restored to her diet foods which we had eliminated, that milk and wheat brought back her symptoms. I told her that, hopefully, after she got on the far side of menopause it might be that she could once again tolerate these foods, although in small quantities and less frequently than before. Still, the possibility was good that she could have them now and again, remain symptom-free, and be "her old, sweet self."

There is a strange aspect to the avoidance approach in treating food allergy that we should mention here since it has emotional features. Some patients heartily resent being told to eliminate certain foods from their diet, especially some foods which they prefer above all and which seem to have given them some sort of sense of security over the years. Such patients, especially if they are already emotionally stressed, may feel deprived and hostile. Oddly anough, the food or foods they prefer are often those which cause their allergic symptoms. Treating food allergy is never so simple a business as it sounds. Patients seem to feel that there ought to be a magic medication which they could take that would allow them to remain symptom-free but to continue to eat what their hearts desired. Alas, even the wisest of shamans possesses no such magic potion.

There are two uncomfortable conditions of the gastrointestinal tract that we should mention here in which emotional stress is deemed to play an important role, although allergy's role, if any, is a matter of controversy.

The first, mucous colitis, characterized by weakness, fatigue, nonspecific aches and pains, and diarrhea with the passing of a great deal of mucus with the stool, often presents itself in the company of a nervous and irritable disposition. Personally, I don't find it surprising that the two should go together–colitis and poor disposition—considering the symptoms. The great difficulty is to know which causes what—the disposition the illness, or vice versa. I am sure in my own mind that mucous colitis would not help my disposition a bit, but I suppose that there are some individuals nervous and tense enough to trigger a good case of mucous colitis. While we are not certain what role allergy plays here, we do know that in some cases of mucous colitis, elimination diets bring relief of symptoms with a corresponding improvement in disposition. We can say, I think, that such cases are very likely allergic in origin and that allergy to foods, especially to milk and wheat, can be the cause in at least some cases of this somewhat generalized complaint. A number of allergists have gone so far as to call this gastrointestinal distress "asthma of the bowels," pointing out that both it and asthma often run in the same family. However, many other physicains, psychiatrists in particular, discount the role of allergy, insisting that mucous colitis is entirely psychosomatic in origin. Ah, well, I shall continue to shake my gourd three times, mutter my incantations, lend a careful and sympathetic ear, proffer my wisdom, and prescribe elimination diets and the like with a fairly strong faith that all will be well with at least some of my unhappy patients—if not all.

The second distressing gastrointestinal condition, ulcerative colitis, is even more uncertain in etiology. This can be a serious illness, requiring major surgery on occasion. And it can be severe enough to cause death. Characterized by diarrhea, bleeding, and chronic ulceration of the mucous membranes of the intestinal tract, this extremely unhappy illness is not considered generally to be an allergic disorder, although there are some allergists who insist that perhaps in 10 percent of its victims it is allergic in origin. A few allergists believe that a majority of cases are allergy-caused. We do know that emotional stress plays a villainous role, however; and there also appears to be some genetic factor, for there is a significant occurrence of the problem within families. One of the reasons that emotional factors are considered to be so important is that there appears to be a correlation of the ups and downs of the colitis, its remissions and relapses, with periods of emotional stress. This relationship is so strong that many physicians, especially psychiatrists, deem it a psychosomatic illness and suggest that its victims share certain common characteristics.

In one study of a number of ulcerative colitis patients, it was observed that they shared a low frustration tolerance; seemed to lack a sense of responsibility; were somewhat immature; suffered feelings of rejection, repressed hostility, and anger; and, perhaps most marked of all, possessed traits of obsession-compulsion. The majority were exceedingly neat and orderly, rigid in their morality and behavior, unblessed by a sense of humor, overly conscientious, stubborn, anxious, and timid. In general, they were overly dependent on Mother, who often as not was the dominating figure in the family and in their lives. Father tended either to be weak and ineffective or absent. On occasion he was brutal and threatening to the patient. Since the listing of these personality traits and characteristics is an after-the-fact business, it is by no means certain that they do not arise from the miseries of colitis itself. We should also note the similarity of these traits with those found in asthma and rhinitis patients and those who suffer skin disorders. It is as though these conflicts and characteristics are shared by the ill no matter what their health problem—which seems as good an argument as any against the claim that a specific personality predisposes to a certain type of illness.

There is little doubt that all sorts of emotional stresses are tied up with food and the act of eating. Most people are familiar with the problem of obesity and the fact that eating can offer gratification when other means fail. Less familiar is compulsive starvation, the problem of anorexia nervosa, in which the individual's loss of appetite can transform him into a living skeleton. Even so, when he can barely lift a finger, he will still not eat and will often insist that he is too fat! Both conditions may be glandular in origin, or emotional, and it is often difficult to diagnose which. Other emotional aspects of eating are embarrassment when dining in public or with certain people, i.e., as with maiden ladies who have difficulty putting food in their mouths in the company of gentlemen they find attractive; nervous vomiting, which is said to be motivated by guilt feelings; choking on food and an inability to swallow, which is said to manifest aggressive impulses.

It is certain that the emotions play the role of the heavy in a variety of gastrointestinal problems, allergy included. However, I am firmly convinced that allergy to food may be at the bottom of a good many obscure GI tract troubles and that such a possibility has been generally unrecognized. What we often have dismissed as nerves may well be allergens at work. For one thing, the daily fare we set upon our tables is replete with substances not there 50 years ago, not even 20 years ago. Some of the great variety of additive, pesticide, antibiotic and hormonal residues may be exceedingly allergenic, and a good part of the population may be vulnerable to such things. By the same token, a good bit of what was in food 50 or 20 years ago has been refined out of existence, which may not be too much help for our nervous systems. It bears pondering.

13

Allergy of the Nervous System

In the *Anatomy of Melancholy,* Robert Burton, a seventeenth century vicar endowed with a large curiosity bump, writes: "That which Pythagoras said to his scholars of old, may be forever applied to melancholy men . . . eat no beans."

Beans! Can they make us melancholy?

In truth, they can. What we eat may depress us, and not just because the cook goofed or the butcher slipped in a tough cut. In fact, what we breathe may also depress us, and not simply because you could cut the smog with a knife. What I as a doctor prescribe by way of medication or injection can also affect not only the mood and emotions of my patients but their behavior as well, and not simply because I have prescribed mood-altering drugs.

How come?

The central nervous system, like the gastrointestinal tract, like the respiratory system, like the skin, is subject to the allergen-antibody battle of an allergic reaction. The results of such reactions can be startling sometimes. Yet in spite of wise Pythagoras and equally wise Robert Burton, and many another perceptive physician and philosopher of old, we have only recently begun to realize the possibilities such allergy may have in the realm of behavior and emotional disturbances. We can only speculate as to how many patients have been dismissed as neurotic in the past when they complained of such generalized and nebulous symptoms as feelings of weakness, extreme fatigue, nervousness and tension, headaches—complaints that cannot be transferred to a microscope slide, cultured in a petri dish, investigated in blood and urine samples, palpated by the fingers, heard through a stethoscope, or seen by the eye.

We can only wonder how many of these ambiguous symptoms *were* caused by an allergic reaction in the nervous system. The number may be legion!

Many an allergist has been somewhat startled to find that when he has brought relief to a patient from such symptoms as asthma or rhinitis, urticaria or gastrointestinal upset, he has also seemed to have relieved his patient of his case of "nerves." Treatment of the obvious allergic problems has diminished the "hidden" allergic symptoms. Allergist and patient alike are astonished at the latter's suddenly altered behavior and/or personality, his abrupt release from neurotic tendencies. For example, we may discover the irritable, fault-finding husband who has berated and terrorized his family into a state of catatonia suddenly transformed into a pleasant, compassionate gentleman when milk and chocolate are removed from his diet.

I believe I now hear the reader clamoring for my attention.

"You mean . . . you are actually suggesting that somebody who acts . . . well, crazy, may simply be having an allergic reaction? May be just allergic to something he eats? Or breathes? Or something?"

Allow me, please, to restate the proposition in my own cautious phraseology. I am saying that an allergic reaction occurring in the central nervous system can give rise to symptoms that can be easily mistaken for neurosis, for mental retardation, and possibly even for psychosis, such states as extreme depression and even characteristics of schizophrenia. We know, for instance, that some cases of epilepsy are allergic in origin. All this is not to say that our mental institutions are chockablock with allergy victims, but only that allergy of the nervous system can create such bizarre behavior and obscure nervous symptoms that superficially we might mistake such allergy for mental illness, and that the more we know about such allergic reactions, the more probable it seems that such mistakes have happened in the past. And may still be happening! Medical specialties still, unhappily, tend to stand aloof from one another. In such matters, closer contact would be reassuring.

And from the reader: "That's strong talk, isn't it, Doc?"

Well, there's nothing like a real-life case to illustrate the point. With his kind permission, I would like to borrow an interesting sequence of events from Dr. William Kaufman, who has written extensively and well on this subject:

Mr. L. was a 60-year-old lawyer. His health had been good until his present illness. He suddenly experienced for a period of four days mental confusion, forgetfulness, and mild ataxia (muscular incoordination). He could not recall what he had done in his office the day before, he found it difficult to express himself verbally, and acted as if he were mildly drunk. He was aware that something was very wrong with him.

As his original set of mental symptoms subsided, he developed considerable fear and anxiety. He thought he had had a small stroke. He did not want to go to his office; he did not want his staff to see him in his weakened condition. And above all, he feared being left alone.

In his office, he cleared his desk of all papers—the "cleaning-up" operation. He wanted his junior law clerks to check his work to be absolutely certain that he made no mistakes. He felt uncertain of his ability to conduct his business competently, and he felt sure that he was not long for this world.

When the cause of his trouble was discovered and proved to him, he became able to function well in his business and elsewhere.

This patient has always avoided eating fruit. Why, he did not know. Occasionally, he did have small amounts without ill effect.

Just before the onset of his illness he had an important brief to prepare, and he did not leave his office for meals. Instead, his secretary brought him lunch, which included 10 ounces of orange juice. In mid-afternoon he had another small meal with 8 ounces of orange juice. The day after this, he experienced the typical primary allergic mental syndrome, which lasted about four days, gradually diminishing in intensity. Before the allergic reaction had subsided, he developed the secondary psychological behavior pattern which was described.

Orange juice was the cause of his allergic mental syndrome. Subsequently, we found that he could tolerate 1 ounce of orange juice without apparent clinical symptoms, but when he had 8 to 10 ounces he had a typical recurrence of his food-induced, allergic mental syndrome. His secondary patterns of unconscious reaction to his allergic illness disappeared with a simple explanation of his allergic illness and the basic psychodynamics of his secondary emotional troubles.*

Dr. Kaufman goes on to explain that a person suffering from such food-induced (or any allergen-induced) mental syndromes doesn't usually realize what is happening to him. Thus he may well believe that he is losing his mind. As Dr. Kaufman says:

he develops unconscious secondary reactions of anxiety, excessive fear of making mistakes, depression, anger with excessive hostile feelings toward

*William Kaufman, *Psychosomatic Medicine,* 16:10, 1954, pp. 29-30.

well persons, with consequential guilt reactions; and he may develop strong dependent needs. Sometimes he may try to deny his illness through excess physical activity. Most often he develops non-problem-solving, obsessive compulsive patterns of behavior.*

The "cleaning-up" act, such as lawyer L.'s desire to clear his desk of papers, Dr. Kaufman calls an avoidance type of behavior, an attempt to bring order to things to help ward off further danger. In children such primary and secondary food-induced mental syndromes can be especially tragic, for the child may carry into adulthood regressive and undesirable behavior and personality traits. The child punished and treated as difficult for a condition he cannot help may be the mentally ill adult of tomorrow. In the hope that it may be of help to other parents in distress, I would like to quote from this sensible letter from Mrs. Myrna Budd of Toronto:

> Our daughter had eczema when only an infant. At seven months she was put on a limited diet of very few foods to control her rash. It worked to some degree.
>
> As she became a toddler, her personality and spurts of energy were almost like Dr. Jekyll and Mr. Hyde. Her rash only came in patches. As a diary of her food intake was kept, I noted various behavioral changes also. As she grew older, her periods of concentration and calmness went from one extreme to another until it finally clicked, and I discovered that when she had foods she was allergic to or was near smoke, she was practically unmanageable or always had tantrums. I began to relate her allergies to her behavior patterns and soon discovered that she was always calm and "normal" when her diet was controlled.
>
> Whenever we visited my in-laws, who are chain smokers, she would always "act up." We finally knew that the combination of "special treats" and smoke were largely responsible for this . . . .
>
> Her facial expression changes and her lips look dry and cracked when she's had too many allergenic foods or is exposed to inhalant allergens. Her personality definitely undergoes a transformation. She becomes restless, looks for trouble, pesty, unhappy, weepy and whiney—generally *ugly.*
>
> Thank goodness we know why now! My doctor still doesn't believe this could happen. But I know it can. I've kept a diary to prove it . . . .

*William Kaufman, "Primary Food-Induced Allergic Syndromes and Their Secondary Psychopathological Accompaniments," presented at First International Congress for Allergy, Zurich, Switzerland, 1951, pp. 972-973.

At least there is one little girl out there who will not be sent warped into the world!

There are many interesting ramifications to such food-induced allergic mental syndromes and their secondary emotional concomitants. We should note, too, that the latter may be an important factor in the emotional stresses that accompany other allergies such as asthma and eczema. We may ask how much of the emotional component that we see with these illnesses is due, as Dr. Kaufman suggests, to ignorance of what is happening to one with accompanying anxiety, depression, and the like—which is not to mention the consequences involved if one's central nervous system is also registering allergic sensitivity!

Dr. Kaufman also makes a distinction between the everyday consumption of an allergenic food, which produces continuing allergy symptoms, and intermittent, occasional consumption. In the first case, he suggests that usually the allergic individual achieves adaption, although neither satisfactory nor efficient, without the secondary emotional syndrome. Such people simply move through their days feeling under par. It is those who suffer intermittent reactions to a food not eaten on a regular basis who may suffer the odd behavior, especially the obsessive-compulsive aspects of the secondary emotional pattern. Such persons, Dr. Kaufman says, occupy themselves with trivia when locked into this pattern, leaving major problems unsolved. With his kind permission, I would like to quote another of his fascinating and illustrative cases here:

> Mrs. J. . . . , a 44 year old housewife told me on her initial visit: "I don't know why, but I get so tired, I just could lay down and die." Physical examination showed no significant abnormality. However, she complained additionally of insecurity feelings because she never knew when she might be sick. She was tense constantly because she feared others would criticize her for inadequacy as a housewife.
>
> Her life was spent planning work in excess of her capacity to do it. She gradually became very busy doing less and less—slower, and much more thoroughly. She kept dusting, cleaning, and setting things in order. If interrupted by a telephone call, she would have to start right at the very beginning and dust and rearrange what she had already completed. She feared making mistakes—often she checked and rechecked her cooking ingredients to be sure that she had not left something out of a recipe. On her so-called good days she undertook excessive physical exertion consisting mainly

of rearranging the furniture. She developed these obsessive compulsive trends in all her human relations, constantly striving for perfection in small and unimportant things while avoiding solution of major issues confronting her as a person.

This case has a nightmarish quality, not only for Mrs. J., but for all who dwelt in her vicinity! Fortunately, there was a resolution of her problems as Dr. Kaufman goes on to explain:

> In this instance, milk chocolate was the offending food. Psychotherapy alone did not benefit her—since her allergenic illness following the intermittent ingestion of chocolate kept recurring as a cue for her unconscious obsessive compulsive non-problem solving behavior. Removal of the allergenic food from her diet alone gave her much relief, with some lessening of the secondary behavior patterns; and with the simple explanation of the dynamics of her emotional trouble and supportive psychotherapy, she recovered completely from her secondary conditioned behavior reactions.*

When we speak of an allergic reaction in the nervous system, what are we saying? What happens?

First, let's identify the parts of the nervous system commonly involved in such a reaction. There are two main divisions of our nervous system: the central, which includes the brain and spinal cord; and the peripheral, which includes the autonomic nervous system and the organs of our special senses (optic nerve, olfactory, and the like). Allergic reactions can occur in both these divisions. The mechanics of what actually takes place is somewhat obscure, but it is believed that vascular changes similar to those that happen in allergic reactions in other body systems, such as hives in the skin, happen in the nervous system also. Such changes, as we have seen, include dilation of blood vessels, leakage of fluid causing edema, and constriction of the smooth muscles. Some researchers believe that an allergic reaction in the cranial area is especially similar to the mechanism of hives. Whether vascular changes can explain all manifestations of allergy of the nervous system is open to question, for we are moving in areas of unexplored territory here. Some researchers, for instance, suggest the mediators (histamine, serotonin) may play a more direct role in the reaction. In general, the effect of

*Ibid., p. 973.

such reactions has been likened to the effect alcohol has on many people. One strange possibility is that allergy of the nervous system can also work in a manner different from any other allergy manifestation to cause demyelination, the degeneration of the myelin sheath of the nerves, such as occurs in multiple sclerosis. Needless to say, this speculation is the object of present research. Also needless to say, there is a great deal about this aspect of allergy that we do not know yet. We suspect much, but our experimental foundation is still somewhat skimpy.

So, then, you ask, how do we know that allergy is at the bottom of neurotic-like symptoms and strange behavior, and headaches?

Animal research in the laboratory has been able to reproduce certain nervous system manifestations. For instance, over 40 years ago, researchers noted that when they induced allergic shock (anaphylactic shock) in rabbits and dogs, brain lesions were found. Experiments with rabbits also demonstrated that antibodies could be produced in the nervous system and that the allergic reaction was not simply a matter of antibodies being circulated via the bloodstream and thus into contact with nerve cells, but was rather a direct confrontation, as it were, in nerve tissue itself.

Among human patients, nervous system symptoms can be elicited by simply exposing the individual to a particular substance to which he has become sensitized. Often other allergy illnesses accompany nervous system symptoms, as we indicated earlier. They can be a big help in diagnosis. However, many allergists now believe that neurological allergic symptoms can stand alone and also that they are far more common than we thought in the past. In fact, an interesting five-year study of nervous system disturbances has turned up some unexpected results. Investigators tabulated patient histories, results of physical examinations, and all signs and symptoms of allergy in hundreds of patients suffering from nervous system disorders and complaints of one kind or another. To illustrate the great variety, I have the permission of Dr. M. Brent Campbell to reproduce this chart of his "Summary of Primary and Secondary Neuro-psychiatric Symptoms of Allergic Origin in a Neuro-psychiatric Population—266 Patients."*

*M. Brent Campbell, *Annals of Allergy,* Vol. 31, October 1973, Table 111, p. 488.

Headaches–allergic or non-specific	90
Mood disturbances	87
Vertigo	57
Gastric symptoms	46
Headaches–migraine	37
Focal or general weakness	35
Focal or general seizures	35
Fainting attacks (blackouts)	30
Minimal brain dysfunction syndrome	28
Myalgia (tenderness or pain in the muscles)	21
Neuritis	13
Numbness	13
Cerebellar	10
Mild periods of disorganization and disorientation	9
Leg spasms	9
Acute or chronic schizophrenia	9
Alcoholism	9
Ocular symptoms	7
Insomnia	6
Sleep disturbance	6
Facial paralysis	3
Stuttering and stammering	3
Autonomic	2
Retrobular neuritis (retrobular meaning behind the eyeball)	1
Jaw spasm	1
Polyneuritic syndrome (inflammation of several nerves)	1

M. Brent Campbell, *Anals of Allergy,* Vo. 31, October 1973, Table 111, p. 488.

Note that mood disturbances–described by Dr. Campbell as "symptoms with psychogenic connotations" and considered by us in this book as emotional stresses such as anxiety, depression, tension, hostility and the like–followed closely on the heels of headaches as the most frequent symptom of nervous system involvement. Dr. Campbell goes on to point out that 87 percent of mood-disturbance patients were allergic to foods, while 22 percent were allergic to dust, pollen, and drugs. In all, of the 207 patients covered fully in this study, 157 proved to be allergic to food, with chocolate and milk heading the food allergen list. It does seem odd to contemplate that eating a chocolate bar now and again can produce excessive anxiety in an individual sensitive to the stuff—or turn on his hostility, or sink him into the depths of depression, sometimes so deep that he may consider suicide. Yet, if he happens to be hypersensitive to chocolate and his nervous system is the body organ registering that sensitivity, his whole personality may be altered by that bar.

Aw, come on, Doc!

Please! Bear with me! Look if you will, for instance, at the following allergic neurological syndrome, called the Allergic Tension-Fatigue Syndrome. I capitalize the title so that it may forever stick in the reader's memory. It may be one of those things he might wish to know sometime in the future—perhaps when confronted by the bizarre behavior of his otherwise charming youngster.

We have heard a great deal of late about hyperactive children, and especially about the controversial use of amphetamines to calm them; for oddly enough tranquilizers only serve to make their overactive condition worse. A good many allergists now believe that some of these overheated youngsters are victims of nervous system allergy. We can't blame all hyperactive syndromes on allergens. Exposure to lead, for instance, may be a large factor in this condition, especially among inner-city youngsters (and adults, for that matter), where lead in the dust and air has increased to an alarming extent. But to illustrate allergy's role, let's construct a somewhat fanciful portrait of a child suffering the allergic tension-fatigue syndrome.

Billy Jones's mother swore that he had not been still five minutes in a row since he was six months old, except when he was immobilized by sleep—which, as far as she was concerned, was not nearly often enough! He had given up naps at six months, depriving his mother of those delightful hours of peace and quiet during which she could recollect her scattered self. Worse still, Billy soon wore out baby-sitters in a ten-block radius, bidding fair to wear out all those in the town beyond. The senior Joneses hadn't taken in a movie in years, much less stepped out to dinner or an evening of bridge. Billy had also long since worn out his welcome at neighborhood kaffeeklatsches, so that the telephone seldom rang for his mother. The home within was also a shambles. Lamps had disintegrated, china was reduced to shards, ashtrays went by the dozen into the garbage can as bits of broken glass, and the TV had twice lost its tube. The truth was, Billy was incredibly clumsy. He stumbled, dropped, knocked into, fell over until he, himself, was damaged, covered with bruises, cuts and scrapes. He was also extremely irritable, and often aggressive. He had made more enemies than friends among his peers.

Alas, nursery school was no solution for his harried mother. The staff, all gentle maiden ladies, would never be the same again. Well, at least, when he arrived at six, the public school would have to accomodate this strange, restless, clumsy, hyperactive boy. That was the law and the school complied. Three teachers resigned not long after to take up less remunerative tenures in private schools not required by law to deal with the undealable. One principal decided that it was time to retire. For several years, Billy roamed classroom aisles, seldom making use of his desk, talking ceaselessly and out of turn, interrupting lessons and lectures alike. By fits and starts, he was moved slowly up through the elementary grades, repeating several on the way–although it was obvious he was no dullard. It was not his intellect that was at fault. He simply could not keep his restless mind on anything.

Nor could he hack it in sports when he tried to please his father by going out for baseball.

"I'm sorry, Mr. Jones," the coach explained as tactfully as he could, "but to put it bluntly, Billy's all thumbs and ten feet, and he can't seem to concentrate for two seconds on what he's doing. Not only that, but he never stops talking long enough to listen to instructions. Worst of all, he takes a hefty swing at a nice easy pitch and slings the bat. I thought he'd broken one kid's shinbone the other day. I hate to say it, but he's a menace out there, a one-kid disaster!"

Well, perhaps we shouldn't make light of so serious a business, for this whole affair was an unhappy and traumatic experience for one small boy and his worried parents. Still, since all stories should have a happy ending, let's tack on one here. The family physician, when finally appraised of Billy's peculiar problem, responded like the wise shaman he was. He checked Billy out thoroughly, then recommended an allergist.

"It may not be the answer," he warned the Jonses, "but I did read an AMA paper in the *Journal* just the other day that was all about steamed up behavior like Billy's. The author believed that a good bit of this kind of thing stems from an allergy to food. So, let's let the allergist have a go at it. Can't hurt and might do you all a lot of good."

"You mean, everything, all this . . . it could just be because of something he eats?" Mrs. Jones was flabbergasted.

"Could be."

And so it was. Billy turned out not be an an original Peck's bad boy after all—after all those years barren of baby-sitters, kaffee-klatsches, and parental pride! And all because Billy was allergic to chocolate and milk, his two very favorite foods, which he, like an older alcoholic, loved too well. Once these foods were removed from his diet, Billy became a different youngster. His whole personality altered abruptly. Oh, yes, he had his peccadilloes like any other ordinary human being, but he became good-natured and almost agile. He began to bring home decent report cards indicative of concentration and of his innate ability. He began to entertain batches of friends, all of whom were given to wearing muddy sneakers. He even asked a girl to a party and, wonder of wonders, he made the baseball team, for at last he had learned how to hang on to the bat!

All this is very strange, you say? Ah, but we have only looked at half the picture. Bobby Brown, who lived half a block down from Billy Jones, presented an excellent foil for his overactive classmate. Pale and listless, Bobby was easier to have around except that his parents and teachers alike found such overwhelming fatigue and unhappiness downright annoying. "Snap out of it, son!" his father would cry, while his mother would sigh and wearily coax, "You can do it if you'd just try, Bobby." But apathetic he stood or sat upon the edge of all activity. It was all he had done from infancy, even though his anxious mother plied him with vitamins and cod liver oil and his father had done his best to make a "real boy" out of his torpid son, buying him an assortment of expensive sporting equipment that gathered dust in the boy's closet. Worse still, Mrs. Brown daily faced the herculean task of getting him out of bed in the morning and properly on his way. Even though Bobby went to bed far earlier than other youngsters his age, and even though his sleep appeared normal, he could not seem to wake up in the morning. Half drugged with sleep, he often had to be driven to school since he habitually missed the bus. And in the classroom he either openly slept or daydreamed his education away. Thus, he, too, advanced through the elementary years in fits and starts.

The same wise general practitioner who sent Billy Jones to an allergist came to Bobby's rescue earlier in the game, mainly because Bobby's problem showed its true colors—or, rather, lack of color, for Bobby was obviously pale and ill-looking. In this case, too, when no physical cause could be found for his symptoms, the doctor advised that an allergist be consulted.

The moment Bobby walked into the allergist's office his problem was partially solved. Bobby sported recognizable symptoms of allergy—pallor, dark circles under his eyes called allergic shiners, narrow nose, somewhat flattened cheeks, and protruding teeth—all characteristic of long-term allergy. This appearance, called the allergic facies, is quite prominent. Like Billy Jones, Bobby turned out to be allergic to food. In his case it turned out to be wheat and corn; thus, his daily breakfast was robbing him of strength and happiness. Once wheat and corn were removed from his diet, Bobby also underwent a change of personality and even a change in appearance as color came back to his cheeks and the dark circles faded from beneath his eyes. Activity and pleasure in life added muscle and flesh to his once puny physique. No dullard, he too began to bring home good report cards and, no longer an outcast, boy friends and girl friends. Happy endings abound in the practice of allergy!

I have separated these symptoms to indicate more clearly the personality and behavior patterns that can develop in allergy of the nervous system; but, in truth, both sets of symptoms often occur in the same individual. Hyperactive symptoms frequently alternate with those of fatigue. Hence the name: allergic tension-fatigue syndrome. Children usually express these tension-fatigue symptoms in their actions and appearance, but adults, too, may clearly indicate their restlessness and/or fatigue. The reader has probably known someone who cannot seem to relax, who, when seated, must shift about in the chair, tap his feet, drum on the table, play with keys or small change, and the like. Such folk sometimes have difficulty finishing a sentence. Although they tend to talk a great deal, they rarely seem to listen. Insomnia is frequently a complaint of the hyperactive, as is that strange business of "restless legs," which can literally drive the sufferer up and out of his bed even though he is dead-tired. Only the legs seem to want to go! The fatigue side of the syndrome seems commonly to appear in adults as irritability and lethargy. Like their young counterparts, they have to drag themselves out of bed in the mornings, and although they have had their eight hours or more of sleep, they often do not feel rested.

Adults, who have an easier time of communicating their feelings and sensations, speak of being jittery, up-tight, jumpy, uneasy, worn-out. They complain of being able to fall asleep at bedtime readily enough, only to wake a few hours later to hear the clock strike every hour until dawn, at which time they fall asleep again just in time to be awakened by their insistent alarm clock!

Like his young counterpart, the adult allergic tension-fatigue sufferer is clumsy and accident prone. He not only gets hurt more than most people, but he hurts himself continually. He is a menace at parties and never to be trusted with the last of the Limoges or Dresden plates.

There are some strange sidelights to this syndrome and to allergy in general. Allergic youngsters and adults alike tend to be overly reactive in what they do and how they feel. You could almost say that this is a personality trait they share. For instance, they are often hypersensitive to noise. Allergic children commonly clap their hands over their ears during a TV western shootout, although they continue to watch with avid interest as good guys and bad guys fall in windrows. Such patients are frequently overly sensitive to cold, heat, light, smells, and pain. It is thought, for example, that their body temperature regulation is faulty or functions poorly. In one study, allergic children asked to hold an ice cube in their hands dropped it in about 20 seconds, complaining that it hurt, whereas nonallergic children were able to hang on to the cube almost a minute. As an ardent tennis buff I have encountered a few people on the courts who actually suffer painfully from the brightness of the sunlight. On several occasions, especially when I have noticed the presence of other allergy signs, I have recommended that they consult an allergist, not to drum up business as the reader might slyly think, but because such painful hypersensitivity to light can be an allergy symptom. Odors, too, are often keenly offensive to allergic individuals. They may smell and rue what others never notice. Perhaps this may superbly equip them as ad-writers for deodorant soap and mouthwash blurbs, but it must be intolerable on occasion. All in all, the world impinges powerfully upon allergic persons. They, in turn, are likely to react more violently than the nonallergic.

Because the tension-fatigue syndrome may be present in one degree or another in much of severe allergy, it would seem logical to suggest that at least part of the emotional stresses that accompany such allergies may be due to actual allergic reactions taking place in the nervous system itself. The following bizarre behavior could be exhibited:

mental dullness	mental confusion
feelings of unreality	delirium
agitation	excitability
impulsiveness	talkativeness
mild mania	yawning attacks

But allergy of the nervous system doesn't stop there. It can cause other disorders that mimic functional neurological diseases. Called a variety of names—"nervous storms," "ecological mental illness"—these conditions still present a good deal of mystery. They not only include Dr. Campbell's long list of neuropsychiatric symptoms, but they can be such as to be mistaken for psychosis. For example, earlier in this book we discussed conversion hysteria and how some young paratroopers of World War II escaped overwhelming anxiety by unconscious paralysis of a limb, usually a leg, and that such paralysis could be so "real" that pins stuck into the affected limb were not felt. Now and again, nervous system allergy can mimic such a state.

Another allergic nervous system syndrome results in muscle weakness that has sometimes been mistaken for myasthenia gravis, an often progressively fatal disease. Another syndrome, Meniere's disease, characterized by dizziness and loss of balance coupled with nausea, frequently is allergic in origin. One of the most interesting findings is, as we have noted, that some epilepsy appears to be an allergic reaction in the nervous system. What complicates this suggestion is that allergy and epilepsy are often found in the same patient, so that the question arises of which causes what. Some studies have indicated that allergic children may have abnormal electroencephalograms (brain wave tracings), but the matter is still disputed.

We can accept with certainty the fact that allergy and neurological disorder go hand in hand, even though we do not as yet understand the mechanism, the how's and the why's. There is a recent alternative hypothesis to the now somewhat accepted role of allergy in nervous symptoms that postulates that such neurological disorders are caused by brain unjury of some sort, which may itself be the cause of the allergic disorders. This theory suggests that disorganization of the nervous system allows the expression of a genetic weakness or vulnerability such as allergy, and that that vulnerability then expresses itself in turn in allergic, vascular, or behavioral disorders.

As you can see, we have here another potential storm center of controversy! But let us devote more space to several still somewhat mysterious aspects of nervous system disorders, especially those involving headaches and schizophrenia and their possible relationship to allergy.

14
Allergy as a Factor in Headaches and Schizophrenia

By now it should be obvious to the reader, or so I hope, that it behooves us shamans to investigate the allergy possibilities in many obscure nervous system and behavioral disorders. It may well be that the oddball friend of ours who drinks beer with gusto and then goes berserk is actually allergic to the molds and yeasts he is quaffing. His brew is literally going to his head, and in more ways than one. We can comprehend, too, I think, why the problem brat just down the block should never let chocolate or cow's milk pass his lips! And why our friend's depressed and complaining wife should never eat wheat in any form so that she might enjoy life again. Thus, it is easy to designate certain behavior as "personality traits," but in truth such traits may simply be symptoms of allergy. Not only do nature and nurture shape us, but nervous system sensitivity may help determine what sort of person we are, at least temporarily. We do know that serious disease can alter personality. In fact, an abrupt change in an individual's character may be heralding a severe illness of some kind, such as cancer. All of which seems to enlarge the question mark punctuating the chicken-egg question—which comes first, allergy or emotional stress?

You aren't totally convinced that all this is so?

Dr. Lawrence D. Dickey of Fort Collins, Colorado, has sent me a number of interesting cases along these lines. With his kind permission I would like to reproduce one here to illustrate such mood and personality changes.

> Mrs. P. F., age 32, . . . first visited this office . . . [in] 1974. Chief complaints were vertigo, headache, and memory problem. She was admitted to the Poudre Valley Memorial Environmental Care Unit on the same day.

She was brought to the office during her hospital stay for inhalant, food and chemical testing. After several food tests, which proved negative, a provocative test for beet sugar was carried out.

Within a minute after being given .05 cc of #1 dilution sublingually (placed beneath the tongue), she began sobbing hysterically. It appeared as if someone had presented her with bad news. The patient was immediately given .05 cc of #3 dilution and within three minutes she stopped sobbing and was still crying quietly. Then .05 cc of a #5 dilution was given and within two minutes she was calm and had stopped crying. Within ten minutes the patient was talking and laughing with other patients. After waiting for twenty minutes she was completely relieved and sent back to the hospital. The patient stated she felt better than she had felt in many years and was quite happy to find a cause for her depression.*

Now if we turn again to Dr. Campbell, we find that he has compiled a descriptive classification of severe allergic reactions in the nervous system that should dispel any doubts the reader may have that such reactions can cause personality changes. With Dr. Campbell's permission, I quote his list:

Emotional Immaturity Reactions:

Included under this heading are temper tantrums, screaming episodes, whining, impatience, and excitability. Patients of this type are inclined to be erratic, impulsive, quarrelsome, and irresponsible. Many admit having "childish" compulsions.

Antisocial Behavior:

These patients are inclined to be uncooperative, pugnacious, sulky, and, perhaps, cruel. Most have learned enough self-control to avoid serious aberrations of behavior.

Depressive Symptoms:

Under this heading are such complaints as inability to concentrate, semi-suicidal ideation, insomnia, worry, and less interest in work and recreation.

Anxiety:

More than is true of patients with simple allergic tension, these individuals are unusually fearful, worried, oversensitive, and restless. Severe nightmares are common.

Organic Brain Syndrome Reactions:

Common complaints are mental confusion, tardiness of thought, stuttering, dullness, partial blackouts, sleepiness, stupor, and lowered mentality.

*Lawrence D. Dickey, M.D., Fort Collins, Colorado.

A picture very similar to hypothyroidism (deficiency in thyroid gland secretion that results in lower metabolism and sometimes cretinism) is common.

Schizophreniform Reactions:

Common manifestations are mild manic excitability, mental confusion, ambivalence, feelings of unreality, dream states, and hallucinations. Short-term reactions occur which simulate classic schizophrenia, but remission is common, especially under allergic treatment.

Habit Reactions:

Marks, in discussing oral habits of allergic children, describes various habits which can be construed as being related to neuroallergy. He mentions sucking the cheeks, lips and tongue; tongue biting; and chewing habits of the lips. Other mannerisms that are seen in allergic patients are neck stretching, yawning, eye blinking, leg and foot tapping, and scratching.*

Hmmm, what else is there?

Well, there is still that cross of all mankind—headache. There are a variety of headaches, but three main divisions are generally accepted—vascular headaches, muscle contraction headaches, and headaches that combine the two. What has allergy to do with this all but universal pain in the head? Probably quite a bit, especially in the case of chronic vascular headaches.

The mechanism of vascular headaches of the migraine type involves disorders in cerebral circulation. The headache begins with blood-vessel constriction, followed by marked dilation. During the constriction stage there may be mood or motor or sensory disturbance to warn the victim that the dilation stage is coming, bringing its throbbing and pain in tow. Visual warnings can be such things as zigzag patterns, like lightning striking through the sky, or flashing lights, or even patches of darkness. Motor signs may be fatigue and muscle weakness. Depression or anxiety may warn of the coming storm. Such signs, called prodromes, usually precede the headache pain by one or two hours. When pain does arrive it may be accompanied by nausea and vomiting and a strong desire for darkness. The migraine type of vascular headache may last anywhere from several hours to several days. It is usually recurrent, the onset gradual, and the pain throbbing.

*M. Brent Campbell, "Allergy and Behavior: Neurological and Psychic Syndromes," in *Allergy of the Nervous System*, ed. Frederick Speer, Springfield, Illinois: Charles C. Thomas, 1970, pp. 31–32.

A second type of vascular headache called the cluster headache differs somewhat from the above description. It comes on suddenly and lasts anywhere from just a few minutes to a few hours. Sometimes called a histamine headache, unlike migraine it can visit its victim at night, bringing him bolt upright from a sound sleep and driving him out of his warm bed with its unbearable pain. The relationship of allergy to this strange head pain that comes in clusters is not so clear as it is in some migraine-type vascular headaches.

There are, of course, other causes than allergy for vascular headaches, some of them serious. These possibilities must be ruled out before allergy can be ruled in. Even then, a variety of other factors—physical agents such as cold, heat, or light; infection; gastrointestinal upsets; and emotional stress—may be so intertwined that the allergic reaction itself is a secondary cause. For example, headache is frequently a symptom of allergy whether it is reasonably mild or of the painful migraine type. When sensitivity to an allergen is at the root of the headache, a number of other factors are usually clear: a family history of allergy, accompanying additional symptoms of allergy; relief of symptoms by antiallergy treatment, be it by avoidance measures, elimination diet, desensitization, or medication.

The following case illustrates an allergy-induced headache pattern with, as far as I could tell, no real emotional stress involvement:

The patient, a forty-three-year-old male, gave a lifelong history of headaches and stated that for the past three years his headaches has become extremely severe. He said that the pain was definitely worse in the late evenings (circadian rhythm?) and that it occurred on an average of "50 to 60 times" a week. The headaches lasted from 10 to 15 minutes, then cleared, but would often recur within 30 minutes.

The patient described the headaches as being "unbearable," and he stated that the pain was located in the left temple region and was associated with nausea. He said that he had been hospitalized in 1973 for a neurological work-up and had been told that he had an "abnormal brain wave." He explained that at times he experienced a "popping and cracking noise" in the roof of his mouth and that when this happened, his headache would be relieved.

He stated that within 30 minutes of drinking beer, he would have a headache and that his headaches were much worse during March, April, and August. They would then decline in severity after the first frost. (All this, of course, provided me with any number of clues: yeast in beer, pollen during the spring and summer months.)

The patient gave a lifelong history of nasal congestion. Rainy weather aggravated it, and he said that he breathed through his mouth and snored considerably at night. He added that he also experienced some tightness in the chest and smothering, and that he was "out of breath" most of the time. Alas, he confessed that he smoked two to three packs of cigarettes a day and had been doing so since the age of fifteen.

He provided further clues to his headache problems when he told me that there were a few potted plants in the house and a dog and cat that lived in close proximity near his bedroom window. He also told me that he had recently acquired a feather pillow.

Answers for this particular patient lay in eliminating some foods from his diet, moving the doghouse from the neighborhood of his bedroom window, giving away the feather pillow to a greatful, non-allergic recipient, putting the potted plants in the garage, and an awful struggle to cut down, if not cut out, those cigarettes. As I said earlier, I could find no emotional overlay to his problems. Allergy was at the root of his headaches.

Far less clearly allergic in nature are muscle-contraction or tension-type headaches. This type of headache is usually in reaction to emotional stress. In fact, many physicians believe that about 90 percent of all headaches are psychogenic in origin. Perhaps for this reason, shamans of various stripes had good luck with their headache patients when they advised that the sufferers should cover their heads with potatoes, bathe their feet in a concoction of mustard and farina, or eat green onions—all of which must have been somewhat reassuring to the troubled headache victim. Such remedies would at least divert the patient from his emotional distress momentarily. The emotion most commonly associated with tension headaches (which are characterized by a dull pain and a sense of pressure and of tightness) is depression. Such headaches occur almost daily and are frequently worse during holidays and weekends, as though the patient found these the most depressing of times. The aching head is usually worse in the mornings and associated with sleep disturbances. Depressive headaches are frequently not relieved by aspirin or other pain-killing drugs, but antidepressants may help.

How does the wise shaman distinguish psychogenic headaches from those caused by definite physical problems or allergy? Once again the patient's history plays a vital role, although physical and neurological examinations are also required to rule out other possibilities such as sinusitis, eye strain, infected teeth, tumor, fever, septicemia, and the like. As he asks his questions about headache symptoms—the location of pain, when headaches occur, what other symptoms such as nausea may accompany them—the wise shaman will mentally note his pateint's appearance and facial expressions. The depressed individual often mirrors his feelings by appearing either very sad or very lethargic and expressionless, as though nothing could possibly make any difference to him any more. His clothing and the manner in which he sits or stands may indicate his despair. He may be untidy and slouching, or, oddly enough, he may be too neat, too rigid.

Headache can also be a symptom of conversion hysteria, becoming an "escape mechanism" for some, just as the paralyzed leg became an escape mechanism for the anxiety-driven paratroopers we discussed earlier. Often such an individual appears immature, anxious, possessed by feelings of failure.

Chronic headache, it is said, also may be a symptom of extreme hostility or aggressive feelings. Headache becomes an outlet for suppressed anger. Or it may be an attention-getting mechanism.

Now, of course, almost all of us at one time or another, and sometimes even rather frequently, suffer from tension headaches. We take aspirin and go to bed a bit earlier than usual, and generally that is all there is to it. Perhaps the next morning dawns more cheerily and we have put our temporary problems behind us. But the patient suffering chronic, recurring tension headaches needs a bit more than this. Mild tranquilizers in combination with antidepressants may be the answer for some as far as medications go, but perhaps the most important ingredient in treatment lies in the physician's relationship with his emotionally stressed patient. Talking out the stressful problem may be a vital part of the "cure."

When we come to a combination of the two types of chronic headache—vascular and tension—we may really have a puzzle. Such a contingency, and it is probably a fairly frequent one in recurrent headaches, really puts the wise shaman on his mettle. How much of the problem is due to allergy and how much to emotional stress?

A wise shaman will now have to admit that a vast mystery still surrounds the whole subject of headaches. It may not be too difficult to improve matters for the purely allergic patient once his allergen or allergens are discovered. It may not even be too difficult to improve the lot of the victim of the tension-type headache once you discover the cause of his emotional stress. But the individual suffering both types, with allergy and stress working together, will surely be a tougher nut to crack. The shaman will no doubt have to resort to every gourd rattle, chicken feather, and dried toad skin in his satchel. To complicate his task, there are all those other "trigger" factors–the presence of infection, weather change, hormonal imbalance, overexertion, and the like. What he looks for is a pattern. Like a police detective studying the MO–mode of operation–of a band of bank robbers, he looks for clues that will predict or identify allergic and/or emotional components. Trying to separate the two is difficult since headaches can affect the emotions even as the emotions can bring about the headaches. It may well be that the wise shaman will also have to determine to what uses the headache patient puts his pain. Headaches have been used so freqnently to duck out of responsibilities and the like that they have become somewhat of a standard joke. And then, you know, such things as sleeping on hair curlers or wearing new bifocals can produce headaches of some potency! Those clues the shaman must seek turn up in odd places!

Is there a headache personality?

Some physicians swear that the tension-type headache, with or without allergic vascular accompaniment, appears in a recognizable personality. He is a very competitive person, a perfectionist, rigid in behavior and morality, who strongly represses hostility and hankerings for dependency. He frequently, they believe, has problems in the sexual aspects of his life.

I, myself, am unsure about there being such a headache personality, but I am sure that a good many headache sufferers owe their pain to "hidden" food allergy and that if they and their shaman have the patience to track down all the clues, they will sooner or later find the villain and exorcise it completely. In the long run it will be a surer cure than aspirin. I believe that most headaches are not mere "nerves," but that "nerves" can make them worse. Therefore, I believe that both sides of the street–allergy and emotional stress—should be worked thoroughly. That, once again, is the concept of holism.

There is another type of patient who frequently complains of recurrent headaches—the schizophrenic. Schizophrenia has presented the medical profession with a first-class mystery for many years. Psychiatrists and other physicians have struggled to find an answer for this tragic disorder, which has afflicted some 2 percent of our population at one time or another. All sorts of research projects are under way at the moment, and some of the leads recently developed appear to show promise. Still, at the moment we have to admit that we simply do not really understand the problem.

One of the great difficulties is that schizophrenia is a label stuck on such an ever changing, complex set of symptoms that it is hard to pin down as a defined condition or disease. It is quite possible to have a ward full of diagnosed schizophrenics with scarcely any two of them suffering identical symptoms.

The schizophrenic individual operates from a reality quite different from the reality the rest of us perceive; thus, he is out of step. His perception of things and people is based on illusion. While he is often quite aware that his perception is faulty, he is helpless to alter his view of life. In his distorted world, he frequently suffers from a terrifying loneliness. No one can see what he does or comprehend what he knows. Because he is often aware of the loss of reality, he may feel cut off and bewildered, and very much afraid of the illusions his mind creates, for these transform the ordinary into the cruel and threatening. His terror may cause him to withdraw from others, even to become almost catatonic, afraid to move or to speak. Or it may cause him to become nervously alert, wary of everything and everyone around him, constantly agitated, afraid to sleep or to rest, lest whatever his mind creates as a threat should attack him.

The schizophrenic's disordered thinking may include hallucinations and an inability to communicate clearly to others. Often it is difficult for him to hang on to the thread of one idea or thought. Rather, his mind overflows with a jumble of ideas, none of which he can unscramble from the others to complete. Thus, when he talks, he pours out this disconnected pile of irrelevant words, completing no formed thought. Obviously, his listeners have a pretty hard time of it. Rather naturally they soon give up, which often makes the schizophrenic frantically try harder. Frustrated, he tries to make order where no order exists.

The schizophrenic hasn't "gotten it altogether," as the young are fond of saying. His "head isn't on straight." In fact, schizophrenia can affect all aspects of the individual's personality. His whole being registers his disorder. The strange thing is that he can act quite normally some of the time, which may be why the idea of schizophrenia as a "split personality" arose. In fact, in times past this apparent normality at one time and obvious disordered behavior at another was cause enough for others to believe him either possessed by the Devil or else in possession of magical powers. It may well be that many an early shaman was in actuality a schizophrenic!

For a long time, schizophrenia was believed to be an inherited mental weakness and incurable. Nowadays, however, we have broadened our view of this strange malady. We believe that there may be multiple causes for the condition, that it is treatable, and that it is frequently curable. While there may be an inherited tendency to schizophrenia, as there appears to be to allergy, a number of recent studies, especially those involving twins, have concluded that the disorder itself is not a genetic trait. No genetic marker has ever been found. Researchers have cautiously advanced the position or theory that a predisposition to mental illness may be an inherited weakness, but most are unwilling to say that this predisposition or tendency is specifically to schizophrenia. Here, I believe, is where the matter rests at present.

In a way, this sounds like very much the same sort of stand we allergists take. We believe that there is a genetic tendency, but we also believe that it is not the only factor at work in the production of allergy illnesses, that the inherited tendency works in conjunction with a number of other equally important factors eventually to produce symptoms. Like allergy, schizophrenia possesses many facets. For example, there is apparently some correlation between schizophrenia and poverty, between schizophrenia and family circumstances that present inconsistency in treatment of the individual during childhood with alternate rejection and smothering affection (somewhat similar to our discussion on asthma), and perhaps between schizophrenia and poor prenatal and infant nutrition. Some researchers have eagerly sought a biochemical cause. One of their hot pursuits has been that of the "pink spot." In the urine of those who are severely schizophrenic there is apparently a compound which produces a pink spot when chemically analyzed. It has been hypothesized that this substance may have hallucinogenic properties. However, there is still a lot more to be learned about the "pink spot."

What has schizophrenia to do with allergy of the nervous system? Well, for some time now, a few allergists have conjectured that something in the environment, something inhaled or ingested, could be causing nervous system sensitivity reactions with schizophrenic-type symptoms, if not some full-blown cases of schizophrenia. Results of a recent study, published in *Science,* 30 January 1976, conducted by two researchers, Man Mohan Singh, M.D., and Staley R. Kay, M.A., tend to support, at least in part, this possibility. The two investigators followed an earlier suggestion by Dr. F. C. Dohan of the East Pennsylvania Psychiatric Institute that there appeared to be a genetic link between schizophrenia and celiac disease, an intestinal disorder that commonly includes an intolerance to wheat and other related cereal glutens. Some patients suffering from celiac disease have been known also to exhibit schizophrenic behavior. In fact, such behavior has often served to help in the differential diagnosis of celiac disease from such other malabsorption and malnutrition conditions as ulcerative colitis. Gluten is known to be a potent allergen; however, gluten intolerance is not actually an allergic reaction but, rather, is akin to the lactose intolerance that is apparently a genetic trait—one's heredity has simply not provided one with the proper enzymes to digest gluten (or the lactose in milk). However, some allergists believe that there is a relationship between gluten intolerance and gastrointestinal allergy. Certainly those who are allergic to wheat and those who are intolerant to wheat gluten must follow the same sort of avoidance diet to maintain their health.

In any case, to find out what sort of influence wheat gluten had upon schizophrenia, Singh and Kay selected 14 schizophrenic patients for their study. The 14 were kept in a locked research room and fed a diet that contained no cereals and no milk in any form. During this period of 12 weeks they did receive neuroleptic medications and a special "drink" daily. During the first 4 and the final 4 weeks of the study, this "drink" contained a soy flour base, but during the middle 4 weeks of the test period, it contained wheat gluten instead of soy flour. None of the patients and none of the staff members working with them were aware of the nature of the "drink." Nor did they know what the study was trying to demonstrate. Both a psychiatrist and a psychologist rated the patients' clinical signs and symptoms of schizophrenia during the research, while the ward staff rated them on their daily social behavior.

The results of the study indicated that the wheat gluten "drink" intensified schizophrenic symptoms and decreased the patients' response to neuroleptic medications. The investigators make no claim that wheat gluten alone is responsible for schizophrenia, but they do state that it is their belief that schizophrenia is a condition resulting from biological and psychological factors working together. They are careful to point out that their study does not establish wheat gluten as *the* villain in this strange mental disorder, but only that it may be one of several factors. Because of its probable multiplicity of potential causal factors, schizophrenia is one illness especially adapted to the concept of holism.

As a matter of interest, foods that contain gluten are wheat flour (labeled usually as just plain "flour"), graham flour, gluten flour, enriched flour, and hydrolyzed vegetable protein, often indicated as "hvp" on labels. A host of food products may contain gluten, as a reader of my earlier book, *Coping with Food Allergy** would discover in Chapter 8, "Our Daily Bread." Substitute flours are also provided for those persons allergic and/or intolerant to gluten.

In the preceding chapter we mentioned that allergy of the nervous system that causes functional neurological symptoms has been tagged with a variety of labels, such as "nervous storms" or "ecological mental illness." The latter label is used most frequently by the proponents of the theory that some foods and chemicals in the environment of our daily and occupational lives can cause symptoms of mental illness. Commonly, they define "ecological mental illness" as encompassing behavior and mental abnormalities resulting from exposure to generally nontoxic and noninfectious substances that are essentially harmless to most people. The theory apparently had its beginnings some 30 years ago when it was noted that some patients given food challenge tests developed psychotic and abnormal behavior episodes. Further testing appeared to establish a relationship between certain foods and abnormal behavior and mental

*New York: Quadrangle, 1974.

disorders. Also, it was established that when the diet of these patients eliminated such foods, behavior and mental disorders ceased. It was also noted that when such foods were occasionally ingested, acute episodes often followed swiftly and markedly, but that when such foods were eaten on a regular and frequent basis, chronic, less acute symptoms tended to develop, which were difficult to correlate with the food consumed.

For instance, there is one rather famous case that crops up repeatedly in the literature of allergy. A woman who was in the habit of drinking 40 (!) cups of coffee daily complained of headaches and suffered from episodes of depression, confusion, and amnesia. Hospitalized, she was placed on a diet that removed common allergenic foods. She improved remarkedly, but when beets were served her at one meal, she regressed acutely. Thus it was discovered that all this time she had been sweetening those forty cups of coffee with beet sugar, and this, if you will pardon the pun, had been the "root" of her problem. Frankly, the 40 cups of coffee would appear to me to be enough to make anyone a nervous if not a mental wreck!

We should note that proponents of "ecological mental illness" believe there are other factors besides foods at work in behavior and mental disturbances. Exposure to all sorts of things in the environment—fumes from cars, gas furnaces, solvents, and the like; air pollutants of one kind or another; insecticides; various materials in such things as bedding, carpets; cosmetics; synthetic drugs—can cause mental illness symptoms.

All in all, there is room here for a variety of theories and need for a great deal more research. It may well be that nutritional deficiencies and allergy are closely related as factors in mental and behavior disorders. It may be that there is a genetic malabsorption or maladaption factor in both. It may be that addiction, whether to drugs, to alcohol, or to food as in obesity, has some common relationship to allergy and nervous system disorders. There are a lot of "maybe's" still to be resolved, and all of them open up fascinating vistas.

15

Sail Away, Little Ships

In the *Golden Bough* Sir James Frazer described how certain peoples banished illness from their midst by constructing miniature sailboats, heaping them high with food and other offerings, then launching them with chanted instructions to sail away and take with them the diseases suffered by the tribe. Rather naturally, when other folk found such little ships washed up on *their* shores, they took fright. They would burn the ships at once, which may have been just as well considering that the food and offerings could easily have brought along disease bacteria or viruses. In some cultures, animals served as the vehicle for dispatching disease. Loaded with the ritual food and offerings, bedecked with colors, chickens and goats were driven from infected villages out into the wilds. Hopefully, they took whatever epidemic the people were suffering with them. Goats, incidentally, were heaped as well with the sins of the village and driven into the desert, arriving in our own time as the "scapegoats" for much more than sin.

Would that I could so simply load little ships with my allergic patients' various emotional stresses! I could set them afloat in the French Broad river and warn those downstream to burn them on sight. Or I could heap such emotional disturbances upon the backs of goats and drive them into the mountains that surround my native Asheville to go, as it were, braying into the wilderness.

Ah, well, we can sigh for good old-fashioned simplicity, but that doesn't take care of the problems. So what *does* an allergist do when confronted by a patient so emotionally troubled that control of his allergy symptoms appears well nigh impossible unless his emotional stress can be relieved? Perhaps eight times out of ten he can employ common sense and sympathy to help his patient comprehend his problems and which way he must turn to solve them, as we shall explore in a later chapter. But before we turn to the ordinary, let us touch upon several interesting and even exotic approaches to the problem of stress in the modern world. The reader should keep in mind that I am not talking about treatment for allergy per se, since that is a subject for another book (although I have included a variety of helpful hints for allergy control in the Appendix). We are dealing here with the emotional aspects of allergy, the treatment of stress that can aggravate and prolong allergic symptoms.

When we talk of treatment, most of us think of pills, injections, bitter draughts, and the like; so let us start with medications. There are drugs that can benefit the allergic patient suffering from powerful emotional stress, but there is one difficulty with this approach. For instance, while the cardinal principle in the treatment of allergy is avoidance of that which causes symptoms, there are various drugs employed to alleviate these symptoms, but these drugs do not "cure" the underlying sensitivity of the patient. They may raise his tolerance level to allergenic substances temporarily, but his allergic condition remains. This is also true of the drugs we would employ to ease his emotional stress. They would not "cure" his problem; they would only make it temporarily more bearable. They might also make it a bit easier to find a solution, for there are many times when a patient is simply too strung up, too overwrought for the shaman's wisdom and common sense to get through to him. It is pretty difficult to explore a problem, much less attempt a resolution, when a patient is so tense as to be incoherent.

So, many an allergist finds it prudent in such cases to prescribe a tranquilizer, knowing that it is not a "cure" any more than a placebo would be. Now I know that tranquilizer has become a household word and that we are a gulping as well as a gullible people in such matters. We would rather take a pill than go to the effort of solving our problems. Still, I have had patients so tightly wound up that I had little hope of unwinding them, much less getting them to understand what they must do to control their allergic symptoms. So, I have employed a little pharmacology on occasion. Fortunately, minor tranquilizers such as the benzodiazephines have replaced the not-so-safe barbiturates once so widely used to relax the tense and nervous. Often such mild tranquilizers not only relieve deep-seated anxiety and insomnia but add a placebo effect, giving the patient the feeling that he is being helped. The relaxing action of these drugs often enables patients to talk out their problems. In the case of individuals who cling to their illness as a coping mechanism, such relaxation may give them a chance to gain insight. Oddly enough, many patients seem to react more successfully to tranquilizers when they are unaware that they are being sedated. Thus, I often simply refer to them as just another antiallergy medication.

In actual fact, the antihistamines prescribed for allergy symptoms are themselves mildly tranquilizing in effect. There are times when they are sufficient unto themselves, doing double duty for patient and doctor alike.

We should note, however, that tranquilizers are contraindicated for those suffering the allergic tension-fatigue syndrome. Strangely enough, stimulants such as Ritalin or an amphetamine seem to calm the hyperactive child. These drugs, however, are presently the subject of considerable controversy. In any case, they mask the child's problem, get him out of his parent's hair, turn him into a classroom zombie, and do nothing at all for his underlying difficulty. I personally do not think children should be so drugged. In one study, when a group of children labeled hyperactive were given such stimulant drugs part of the time and placebos part of the time, the investigators had no difficulty identifying the days when the children were under the influence of the stimulants. They became almost emotionless little robots. The sad and even dangerous part in all this is that while such children are being drugged into amiability, their underlying condition, whatever it is, goes untreated. It can be as serious as a cardiac problem or as everyday as allergy to a food. As an example of the latter situation, one doctor has reported a case of a small boy who could not be pleased, who was irritable and restless, a trial to all. When the allergist discovered that tomatoes were at the heart of the matter and eliminated them from his diet, the youngster's personality did a flip and he became a thoroughly pleasant child.

Treatment must also take into account certain "at risk" times in our lives, the phases in our biological rhythms which increase our vulnerability to both emotional stress and illness. Sometimes, for instance, endocrine imbalances which affect our allergic threshold as well as our emotional balance may be corrected by hormone treatment. Adolescence and menopause, for example, are such "at risk" ages.

We cannot put down this discussion of drugs and the emotional aspects of allergy without noting one psychological factor in drug usage. When bronchodilators were introduced into the treatment of asthma some 15 years ago, they were heralded with relief and high hopes. Here was a quick, effective way to head off or relieve asthma symptoms on the spot. These pocket nebulizers could deliver the proper dose of medicine immediately. The patient could do-it-himself as soon as his initial symptoms developed, and relief was prompt. What wasn't foreseen was that asthma patients, terrorized by their attacks, might become so dependent upon their broncho-dilators, some of which contain hundreds of doses, that they would turn to them at the slightest hint of a wheeze. Or even sooner. Soon allergists were worrying about overdosage and overuse, for improperly employed, the nebulizers can intensify asthma symptoms and even cause death. The misuse of such drugs is a clear warning that patients, especially those suffering emotional disturbances either because of their allergy or for other reasons, are likely to use medications as a crutch. Drugs cannot be the whole story in the search for a cure. Opening the medicine cabinet may be a start and often it is a necessary one, but if the patient is to walk and run upright through life rather than stumble and limp, the shaman's draught of wood ashes, toad's blood, and human fingernail parings is only a part of what is needed.

So, what else do we carry in our little black bags?

Well, from time immemorial physicians have shipped their chronically ill patients off to the seashore or to the mountains for the "cure." Since this has been a popular treatment for hundreds of years and since many a resort and spa have grown rich and famous on the sufferings, real or imagined, of these patients, perhaps we must admit that there is some benefit in it. Actually, in the case of allergy there could be—at least temporarily. A change of food, water, atmosphere, climate can mean a change in environmental allergens and diminution of allergic symptoms. Emotionally, too, a change of scene and leaving one's immediate problems behind may help, again at least temporarily. And there lies the fly in the ointment—temporarily. The allergic person remains allergic, and his symptoms will undoubtedly be revived the moment he returns to the old environment. Equally, the emotionally stressed individual would move back into all the old problems that had caused him difficulty in the first place; and unless he was fortunate enough to have gained insight and a solution during his change of scene, he could well find himself in turmoil once more. So, while a vacation, a trip, or a joyride is helpful, it is more likely than not to be a temporary help, not a cure.

There is, however, one factor in such a change of scene or prescribed holiday that may make the difference—relaxation. Relaxation is a key to much of our ill-health and emotional distress. If we could learn to turn that key, we could find our way back to happiness. By relaxation I do not mean that obtained simply by climbing into a deck chair to stretch out in the sun, nice as that can be. To be really helpful, relaxation must be more deep-seated and a more thoroughly learned response than that. We can achieve it in various ways. Tranquilizers, as we just mentioned, are one way. Vacations may be another; but both are, as we noted, likely to be temporary. What we need is a method of relaxation that we can call our own and that we can summon whenever we feel the need of it—a permanent method of relaxing. We also need a deep-seated state of relaxation to dig down to the roots of allergic and emotional problems so that we can expose and understand them.

One somewhat exotic mechanism for achieving such relaxation is through hypnosis. Hypnosis, considered by many to be a kind of nightclub act or parlor trick, is actually a means of inducing an abnormal state of suggestibility in an individual. In some manner not thoroughly understood the reasoning part of the brain is lulled into inactivity, usually at the hypnotist's suggestion that the subject is drowsy, relaxed, sleepy. Some individuals, apparently far more suggestible than most, will fall into a hypnotic state upon a single command or even upon being handed a slip of paper that commands them to relax and feel drowsy. Hypnotic trances can also be self-induced. Fortunately, lest we worry about an absent-minded hypnotist going off about his business leaving any number of people trapped in a trance, the hypnotized snap back into wakefulness in their own good time and on their own.

Ah, but can hypnotism help the allergic patient with an overlay of emotional stress? Can this procedure suggest good health to him, and can we expect it to take? Not, I think, as a general rule. In the majority of those susceptible to hypnotism, the body alterations suggested by the hypnotists appear to revert all too soon to their prior state. In most cases hypnotism does not seem to change the physiological processes for any length of time, the fight-or-flight tension pattern, for instance, which may be aggravating the allergic condition. Like tranquilizers, hypnotism may allay temporarily such emotional stresses, calm the hyperactive patient, and the like, but relapses are frequent, so frequent as to make it a doubtful "cure." In fact, I believe the estimated degree of success runs around 5 percent, and that may be a generous figure.

But hypnotism is nonetheless interesting, so let us explore a little further. There are some strange accounts in the literature of hypnosis. For instance, one subject when touched by a pencil and told that he had been burned, developed a blister at the site. You would think that if hypnotic suggestion could raise a skin inflammation in such a manner it could also banish skin inflammations of various sorts. In fact, a good many experiments to banish warts via hypnosis have been performed, but the results are inconclusive. In one study, for instance, about half the subjects lost their warts after hypnotic suggestion. Interestingly enough, those most susceptible to hypnosis lost theirs the quickest. I suppose the half who retained their warts weren't considered amenable to suggestion. In a later study that attempted to repeat such findings, two groups of subjects with warts on their hands were followed over a period of time. One group was hypnotized and told their warts would vanish within two weeks. The other group was given placebos and told the medication would remove the warts as speedily. Neither group lost warts within five weeks, and, in general, the warts in both groups seemed to follow a wart's natural cycle of apparent self-banishment when they got good and ready.

On the other hand and in all fairness to the hypnotic technique, in studies of known psychosomatic patients (I hesitate over the use of the word "known," however . . .), researchers were able to suppress laboratory-induced eczema in three quarters of their subjects. There is also in the literature the tale of a child known to be allergic to chocolate who under the spell of hypnosis could eat this delight with no adverse effects–hives in his case. What's more, at the suggestion of the hypnotist this youngster could produce hives on one side of his face, then make them vanish at the hypnotist's command.

Such strange maneuvers can be entertaining and mind-boggling. Hypnotism can induce relaxation and convey suggestions of emotional and allergic good health. Probably in some cases it can raise the level of the allergic patient's tolerance to allergens, at least temporarily, by lowering his level of emotional stress. But, as I indicated earlier, I don't believe that it is a generally efficient or permanent attack upon the problem. However, proponents claim that it has had good results on some long-term cases of eczema and other allergic dermatitis conditions. Conversely, they are usually willing to admit that it hasn't been a highly successful therapy for hay fever or asthma.

There is a darker side to hypnosis, a certain psychological danger that should be mentioned. The emotionally overcharged allergic patient who submits hopefully to hypnosis as a cure but finds no relief or else is jubilantly cured only to relapse shortly thereafter may be even further stressed. To be told firmly and commandingly under hypnosis that you would scratch no more, only to find yourself still digging furiously at your skin, could be devastating—especially if you were already excessively anxious or depressed. For this reason, allergists who may turn to hypnosis for help with intractable cases will take care to combine treatment procedures for the allergy itself as well. Do not, we are warned early in life, put all your eggs in one basket!

Some of the most interesting methods for deep relaxation have come out of the mysterious East. It may be that as our technological society becomes more complex and stressful, we, too, are going to have to learn how to control our own physiology to protect it. Both the Yogi of India and the Zen Buddhists have demonstrated that such control of the autonomic or unconscious bodily processes is possible. We have recently become aware that such control may even be essential to good health. There are several variations on the general theme of control of unconscious physiological processes, some of which take a lifetime to master. Few of us have a lifetime to give to it; so we will discuss a relatively simple sort of offshoot that needs only a few training sessions and which can be practiced just about anywhere by anyone—at one's office desk, in bed before rising, even if necessary when stalled in commuter traffic.

Transcendental meditation, called, thank heavens, TM for short, is now widely practiced in this country, and is gaining new converts every day. More importantly, it is attracting scientific and medical attention. Developed by Maharishi Mahesh Yogi, this relaxation technique is taught by a group of trained instructors and even boasts a university, the Maharishi International University in Los Angeles, California. The technique is standard everywhere and easily learned within, according to the instructors themselves, a few hours. The individual then practices the art twice daily for periods of 15 or 20 minutes. As I said, it can be practiced just about anywhere, but the quieter the place and the less distraction, the easier it is, especially for the novice. The subject arranges himself in as comfortable a sitting position as possible, closes his eyes, and lets his mind contemplate a sound, usually a single syllable word such as "love." He does not try to concentrate on this sound, called the "mantra," but he simply lets his mind repeat it over and over. If other thoughts intrude, he switches back to the mantra, although he does not try to force such switching. There are official mantras prescribed by the instructors, but any soothing simple word would probably do, according to some practitioners. Rather naturally, instructors disagree on this. In any case, the more the meditator practices the art, the more adept he will become at reaching a state of deep rest and relaxation. TM is thus a sort of do-it-yourself Yoga adapted to the hectic pace of our western culture where even relaxation must be achieved on the run. It lacks the arduous physical training and postures of more traditional Yoga and does not offer the precise control of autonomic functions, but it does appear to allow the practitioner to attain a high degree of physical and mental relaxation, an end to be greatly desired.

How does it do this? Nobody seems to know for sure. One theory is that the act of thinking of the mantra over and over again sets up vibrations in the nervous system that have a soothing effect. Another theory states that concentrating on a simple word cuts off other thoughts and their related emotional impact. Some simply say that it works a little like a mother singing Brahms' Lullaby over and over again to her child.

However it does what it does, it does do something to the physiology of the meditator and all in the right direction for relaxation. There are several ways to measure emotional stress in the laboratory. One way is to measure skin resistance by taping electrodes carrying small electric currents to the hands. Called galvanic skin response

(GSR, for short), fluctuations in skin resistance are more frequent than normal under the influence of emotional stress such as anger or fear. The rate at which a subject can become habituated to a stress situation can also be measured by such fluctuations. The faster the habituation to emotional stress and the lower the initial fluctuations in GSR, the better the mental health of the subject tested, it is said. So, when two groups were studied, one which practiced TM and one which did not, the results of tests for such galvanic skin response indicated that the meditators in general had lower levels of fluctuations and a faster rate of habituation. Thus, as a group, meditators appeared to suffer less emotional stress than nonmeditators.

The actual physiological changes that occur during meditation have also been demonstrated in the laboratory. Meditating subjects were hooked up to various machines to measure blood pressure, heart rate, skin resistance, body temperature, and brain waves. Oxygen samples were also taken at intervals. It was found that during meditation oxygen consumption diminished significantly, as did the elimination of carbon dioxide, indicating that metabolism was lowered. Blood pressure went down during the resting pre-meditation period and remained down during and after meditation. Heart rate slowed by approximately three beats a minute in the majority of subjects tested. Skin resistance rose, indicating a faster rate of habituation. The electroencephalograph indicated a significant increase in slow alpha waves, the kind of brain wave that all but disappears during mental effort. In general, what appears to happen physically during meditation is the exact opposite of what happens during the fight-or-flight response to emotional stress. The sympathetic nervous system's activities are decreased, including constriction of blood vessels and smooth muscles. Thus, such meditation would seem to bring about the physical alterations necessary to banish *both* emotional stress and allergic reaction. We should also note that laboratory findings indicate that what happens during meditation is quite different from the physical alterations that occur during either sleep or hypnosis. The meditative state is wakeful and aware. Oddly enough, the relaxation it produces is deeper even than that of sleep.

I said a few sentences back that the physical alterations that take place during meditation are opposite to those occuring during emotional stress and allergic reaction. An actual study was made to determine the effect of TM on asthma patients, since such alterations suggest not only decreased oxygen demand but the opposite of the constriction that affects the smooth muscles of the airways and causes pulmonary obstruction. This study lasted six months. The patients were divided into two groups, one that learned to practice TM and the other which was given Maharishi Mahesh Yogi's book *Science of Being and Art of Living.* It should be noted that his book does not tell one how to practice TM. After three months, the two groups of asthma patients switched, and the first group read the book while the second learned and practiced TM. During all this the patients kept daily dairies and records of their medications, answered questionnaires, and had pulmonary function tests made before the study began, halfway through at the time of the switch, and at the end. Such tests measure the degree of airway obstruction in asthma patients. The results were not dramatic and the patients were not "cured" of their asthma; but it appeared, at least from this study, that TM decreased asthma symptoms and airway obstruction. The majority of the patients also *felt* that TM had helped their asthma, and their physicians in answering their version of the questionnaire tended to concur. At the end of a year an additional questionnaire produced the same results: asthma patients considered that TM had helped them, and, again, their doctors concurred.

So, if we have no "cure" here, we may have an assist! Perhaps like the breathing exercises we prescribe for our asthmatic patients, TM can diminish attacks and lower vulnerability. In any case, a technique for relaxation can be of inestimable value in our hectic age!

There are, of course, other means to attain relaxation, and various practitioners swear by their various methods. We must remember too that almost any form of psychotherapy will benefit a good many patients, some say as many as half, simply because of the relationship of therapist to patient. This relationship in itself can reduce anxiety, loneliness, even depression. One form of relaxation, called progressive muscle relaxation, teaches the patient to recognize tension in his muscles so that he can learn to relax them at will. In this method he is told to tense a given muscle to find out how it feels when so tensed; then he relaxes the muscle. In this manner, he learns the difference of feeling in both states.

Debora Phillips, Director of Clinical Training, Children's Program, at Temple University Medical School, explained this technique to me recently:

> The child (and/or patient) is asked to make a fist with his right hand if he is right handed, his left hand if he is left handed. Then he is asked to think about the tension in his hand. After this, he is asked to do the exact opposite of that tension, to relax the hand and to think about how different it feels than when it was tense. He may be asked to raise his eyebrows high with his eyes closed and then to gradually lower his eyebrows so they are relaxed, and to think about smoothing out his forehead. It is especially important for relaxation to take place in the facial muscles and the area around the jaws and throat. The child can be asked to wrinkle up his nose so that he learns what tensing is, and then to relax the nose. He can be asked to make a tense bite with the back teeth, to bite down hard and then relax the jaws, allowing his mouth to remain open a little bit and to think about letting his jaws relax . . . .

Relaxation, however, may be only half the battle. We may need other mechanisms to overcome emotional stress. One interesting procedure is (emotional) systematic desensitization, a process much like the one we allergists use to desensitize a patient to, say, the pollen that is causing his hay fever. We do so by injecting very small amounts of extracts of that pollen initially and gradually increasing the amount until the patient achieves a normal tolerance to the pollen. In much the same manner, a person's tolerance to emotional stress can be raised.

For instance, we know from experience that usually the more we are exposed to a situation, the more skillful and habituated we become in handling it and the less our anxiety is, usually, about it. When one first begins to drive a car, the whole business is pretty exciting and even nerve-wracking; but the more he drives, the less he even thinks about it, and rarely does it thrill him. He can even drive familiar routes without realizing that he has done so. Thus, his anxiety has all but vanished—which sometimes may not be too good a thing. At any rate, desensitization of stressful emotions follows this pattern in a way. The patient suffering from severe anxiety, for example, is told to imagine situations that produce that anxiety, beginning with situations which do not create too much stress for him, then moving progressively toward those that do, once he has mastered the ability to imagine those at the lower level without much ado.

As an example, let us take a woman who has an asthma attack whenever she has to have dealings with her mother-in-law, and who is, in fact, apt to be extremely nervous around any member of her husband's family. Once she has achieved a relaxed state by whatever means—TM, muscle relaxation, tranquilizer, or whatever—she is told to imagine a scene in which her husband tells her he is going to visit his family. She is told to play this inner drama repeatedly until it no longer makes her feel tense. Then she is told to imagine that her husband tells her his sister is coming to their home for a visit, his sister being the least anxiety-provoking member of the family. When she can face this idea without nervousness, she is moved up the scale to an imagined visit from, perhaps, her father-in-law, and so on until she can face the prospect of a visit from or to her mother-in-law without going into an emotional tailspin.

You don't believe it could work? Well, according to its practitioners, it does, and most of the time.

It is possible to transfer the imaginary deed into the real-life situation. For instance, Ms. Phillips, in discussing the case of a twelve-year-old boy with severe asthma whose very fear of his attacks was precipitating them frequently and aggravating their severity, explained the systematic desensitization steps that were taken to diminish both fear and his attacks:

> After we arrived at a list of anxiety provoking scenes, we placed them in progressive order: least anxiety provoking scene to most anxiety provoking scene. While the child is relaxed, he is asked to imagine a scene that provokes anxiety. For example, being sick. If the scene provokes any anxiety, he is asked to stop imagining it and to relax again. Then the scene is presented again. It is presented repeatedly until he can experience it in imagination without having any anxiety. This is what was done with this asthmatic boy. His lowest anxiety provoking item was sneezing, the highest seeing himself in a coffin. Going through these items took eight sessions. At the beginning of treatment his asthma attacks were occurring with the frequency of approximately one every ten days and at the end of treatment they were occurring less than once every two months. And their severity was reduced so that hospitalization was no longer necessary. There was a follow-up of this child (two years later) and the gains were maintained.

Ms. Phillips also discussed relaxation techniques as treatment for headaches—migraine, tension headaches, and the like:

> With the more severe migraine headaches we've had more success combining muscle feedback and relaxation. We focus on relaxation of the frontalis muscles in the forehead, mostly with the raising of the eyebrows and then the gradual lowering of the eyebrows. We ask patients to picture their foreheads becoming smoother and smoother and smoother. We ask them to knit their brows down towards each other and then to relax them. We ask them to close their eyes just tight enough to sense tension, then to release that tension. We use pleasant imagery also—lying in the sun, on the sand, at the ocean, in Barbados, or whatever it is that is relaxing to them . . . .

There are a number of variations on the general theme of relaxation of mind and body, and some control of the autonomic nervous system that all have as their main goal—a reduction of stress and a more successful adaption with a consequent gain in health and happiness. And, as is the way of the world, technology, which has on the one hand so greatly contributed to our stress, has on the other provided instruments by which we can not only measure our stressed condition but also perceive it quantitatively. For oddly enough we are not always aware that we are anxious or depressed, or how badly; nor when such emotions are prolonged, are we aware of the physical alterations they are causing in our bodies. In the last few years the use of biofeedback in relaxation training has taken quantum leaps. New, ever more sensitive machines can now monitor our various physical alterations in response to emotional changes. Hooked to these machines, we can become instantly aware of changes in blood pressure and heart rate, for instance, and thus connect our feelings or sensations of that moment with the physical alterations going on inside our bodies. When we become aware, for example, that fretting over our income tax return raises our blood pressure to an unhealthy degree, we can go about training ourselves to think of more pleasant things.

We in the Western world have come very late to the realization that we *can* control a good bit of our autonomic nervous system once we become conscious of the connection of emotional stimuli and physical response. This ability may be as important in preventing a number of illnesses as was the conquest of disease-producing bacteria or viruses. If rats can be trained to dilate the blood vessels in one ear and not the other, then human beings can surely be trained to regulate their blood pressure. As a matter of fact, with the aid of biofeedback technique, some cardiac patients have been taught to regulate both their heart rate and blood pressure. The instantaneous information provided by various biofeedback tools can accomplish consciousness of the internal self that it takes the Yogi years to master. For instance, one such machine that measures alpha brain waves via the scalp teaches the user how to relax by sounding off through an amplifier when the alpha waves of a relaxed body and mind are achieved. Other machines register the internal states we are not ordinarily aware of with flashing lights or sounds. Thus, we learn to associate certain mental or emotional states with corresponding internal physiological states—the slower beat of our hearts, diminished respiration, lower blood pressure, and the like. In actuality what we learn to control is our subjective feelings which trail the physical changes in their wake, even as we connect feelings of threat or danger with a pounding heart, tightened muscles, increased breathing, and so on.

Once we have made this connection between our emotions and our physical responses, we can begin to retrain ourselves not only to relax but to find more successful ways to adapt to stress. Called behavior therapy, this technique embraces several approaches, one being the systematic desensitization we have already described. Another retraining method called covert conditioning resembles systematic desensitization in that it substitutes an opposing emotion for the one stimulating the adverse physical response. For example, let us take an ambitious young man who wishes to go far in his company, but who develops a splitting headache whenever he must present one of his usually brilliant ideas to his bosses. Tension, anxiety, nervousness—all combine to cause the physical alteration that brings him pain. Why is he so tense then? What is he thinking that makes him so anxious before such presentations? Mostly it seems that he is afraid of failure, that he will botch the briefing, that he will stutter and sweat and make a fool of himself. He lacks, in a word, self-confidence. The solution? He must be retrained to think positively, to imagine himself cool as a cucumber, to imagine that he is presenting his idea under perfect control to men whose faces register instant admiration.

Aha, you recognize something here? You're right—the power of suggestion. But it isn't quite so simple, and it is not something we can learn to do overnight. Habit has a way of becoming deeply ingrained, so that it takes time to root it out and change direction. How is this done? By reinforcement of the emotion we wish to substitute for the young man's anxiety—in this case, self-confidence. Reinforcement can be any sort of positive reward ranging from candy to praise. I suppose in the above young man's case, praise would be the medium.

The marriage of retraining (or covert conditioning or counterconditioning) and biofeedback has produced some interesting results in allergy. Some asthmatic patients whose asthma was initially triggered by infection or allergy become habituated to their attacks because of a variety of stimuli such as weather changes or emotional stress. They respond to these stimuli with bronchoconstriction. It was reasoned that if they could be retrained to respond to these same stimuli with bronchodilation instead, they might well be able to control their asthma or at the very least diminish their attacks. In an interesting recent study, 20 asthmatic youngsters varying in age from eight to fifteen were selected at random from patients at the investigators' allergy clinic. They were then divided into two groups—reactors and nonreactors—on the basis of their responses to inhaling saline vapors accompanied by the suggestion that this substance was a potent allergen to which they were sensitive. The youngsters were then conditioned to respond to suggestion with bronchoconstriction, then trained with the help of biofeedback to replace bronchoconstriction with bronchodilation. When they achieved the latter, a red light would flash on and the experimenter would praise them lavishly. The youngsters were carefully coached in the relationship of the light to their lung function. Thus, when bronchoconstriction was induced by suggestion, the youngsters worked hard to achieve bronchodilation and thereby turn on the red light. In a follow-up study a year later, it was found that the youngsters so conditioned had a greater significant improvement level of their asthma than a control group not counterconditioned. The investigators make no extravagant claims for their work and point out that such conditioning would be an adjunct to the treatment for the allergy or infection that was the basic cause for asthma.

Group behavior therapy, which employs many of the above techniques, adds the stimulus of interaction with others suffering similar problems. It provides the somewhat comforting feeling that one is not alone. There are several set techniques for group therapy, such as psychodrama in which patients act out their problems. Or they may simply be a passive audience while a therapist explains the fundamentals of emotional stress and encourages them in question-and-answer sessions. Usually, group therapy becomes more a talking-out session with the therapist contributing now and again at opportune times. Oddly enough, members of such a group achieve insight into other member's problems before they find their own. Group therapy has only recently been employed for some allergy patients, but has already proved of value for parents of youngsters suffering intractable asthma.

Group therapy is helpful in providing the individual with insight into and expression of his emotional problems. It is hardly possible to cope with something you do not comprehend or are not even aware exists. More than that, it is a truism that bottled-up or repressed emotional stress does the most physical damage. In a study of a number of allergy patients involved in group and individual psychotherapy, it was demonstrated that allergic symptoms and emotional states accompanied each other, but that when the emotional problems were communicated within the group or to the therapist, they became acceptable to the patient, and his allergy symptoms diminished. When he did not communicate his distress, however, his symptoms were retained.

One interesting aspect of group therapy occurs with young children in a form of play therapy. There are a number of variations on the theme of play therapy. We have already mentioned giving youngsters dolls or puppets with which they may act out some of their emotional conflicts. Play therapy may also be an individualistic, child-to-therapist matter; but some recent interesting work has been done with small groups of youngsters. One approach is to have the children play an imaginary game in a magic playroom. Here they turn on an imaginary TV set to the channel that will tell them what problem one of their number, a volunteer, will be working on. The therapist makes sure the youngsters know what this is, then has the volunteer switch to another channel that will show him the same problem that he has had in the past. The other children all act out this problem as the child narrates how it happened to him in the past. He then turns to still another channel in which the therapist and other children reach an understanding of the incident and how it relates to the present problem he is confronting.

Another group therapy program for youngsters (usually up to the age of ten) employs physical-activity games as outlets for emotions such as anger, fear, and grief. For example, bombarding each other with soft plastic balls can arouse and express anger. When the therapist recognizes an emotion surfacing, he stops the game and encourages the children to verbalize and thus recognize their feelings. Children are helped to get out and communicate strong emotions in this manner, which, as we just noted, leads not only to better emotional health but may also assist in alleviating such physical symptoms as allergy.

All of this is very interesting, even heady stuff, but not necessarily within the purview of a busy allergist. Still there are aspects of some or all of these techniques that he and/or his patients may be able to apply, as we shall see as we go on to discuss allergy within the family environment in the next chapter and allergy within the individual's social setting in the chapter after that.

16

Nobody Understands Me!

"Nobody understands me! Least of all my own family!"

My office frequently rings with this sad and plaintive cry, and for the allergic individual there is often truth to it. As we have noted, allergy is so strange an illness that it seems incomprehensible to many people that it could be a real disease. It does not really make much sense that very ordinary things of the environment can affect some people, often violently, and not others. Small wonder the allergic individual finds himself confronted by considerable skepticism and that even his own loving family looks upon him askance upon occasion.

Worse still, allergy can disrupt family relationships, and its presence can transform an ordinarily functioning family into a den of Dr. Bell's attackers and avoiders, pleasers and performers. For some unfortunate allergic sufferers, the family can literally be a hell, and as long as they remain within its circle, they remain chronically ill. This unhappy state of affairs may be due to a number of factors. It may simply be that the home environment abounds with allergenic substances—dust, mold, pollens, feathers, animal danders, and the like. It may be also that the emotional climate within the family is loaded with stress, which in turn diminishes the allergic individual's tolerance to allergens. It may be that his allergy disease in itself contributes to or even causes emotional disturbances among other family members with a rebound effect upon himself, for the manner in which other members of the family respond to his illness may aggravate and increase the severity of his symptoms.

The family, ancient and worthy institution that it is, can be a prime source of ill health and emotional distress.

So, you say, what else is new?

Well, sometimes it pays to comment upon the obvious to ensure that nothing slips by unattended.

We will touch only briefly on the first factor—a home awash with allergens in one form or another. Of course, the outside world is also similarly equipped. Is there no escape? Can the allergic individual turn his castle into a refuge? Yes and no. We'll start with the negative. There is not much the individual family can do about pollution and climate unless it simply picks up stakes and moves to less polluted or allergenic realms. Nor may it be financially possible to build a new or thoroughly renovate an allergenic-type home (such as one with a moldy basement in a damp situation too enclosed by lush vegetation and too close to a busy highway befogged by hydrocarbon fumes). Still, there are many measures we can take to secure the fort, and for the reader's convenience I have listed them in the Appendix:

How to keep an allergen-free house and bedroom, page 225
How to combat mold and mildew, page 228
How to avoid insects if allergic, page 230
How to manage an elimination diet, page 232
How to avoid aspirin-related foods and additives, page 234
How to stop smoking, page 237

Before I begin to delve into family relationships and accompanying emotional stress, I would like to interject here a how-to: namely, how to keep the mother of a chronically ill child from climbing the wall. Mothers tend to be blamed for much these days, yet the burdens of the family and especially of illness in the family rest in the main on their shoulders. In the case of allergy, the mother is the one who must take the extra effort and responsibility for avoidance measures, elimination diets, and the like. And a child or husband who suffers moderate to severe chronic allergy can mean a great deal of extra work for her, far more than many people realize, even doctors. It seems to be imperative that if she herself is to remain emotionally and physically healthy, Mother needs time arranged that she can call her own. If baby-sitters and the like are beyond the family budget, then Father must step in to help. There is no reason why weekends cannot be shared and a good part of one day at least turned over to Mother so that she can get out of the house and away from the problem. She needs very much to be able to walk out of the home, secure in the knowledge that all will be well, and live a few hours just for herself—to recharge her batteries, regain an adult view of the world, or what you will.

I am saying all this so that mothers everywhere will not become totally incensed at what has been said about overprotective and rejecting mothers in this book. As I said, mothers get blamed far more than fathers for the defects we believe we see in the coming generation. Many in the field of medicine have added to the mother's burden of guilt and self-condemnation by accusing her of being the chief cause for her children's emotional disturbances. If this is true, and it may well be, it is possibly because she, also, has suffered emotional deprivation along the way, with her own self-esteem crippled, her own need for independence stifled, her own anxieties intensified.

Having now paid tribute to motherhood, I hope all else here will be forgiven.

Most of the steps we take to reduce allergenic substances within the home have little or no emotional overlay (except for Mother, who must make the effort); but there is one highly emotional problem that keeps cropping up among my patients, especially among my young patients. Perhaps we should mention it here before we go on to discuss family relationships. This is the problem of those allergic to animal danders, and it boils down to one of allergy's severest commandments—No Pets! Furry or feathered, pets give off scales and scurf that are highly allergenic. But, alas, dogs and cats and other furred and feathered companions have a sly way of becoming full-fledged members of the family. They insert themselves with immense cunning, practically seat themselves at the table. Certainly they share beds, meals, and affection. When it comes to banishing them, you might as well draw straws and banish one of the family instead. In fact, many of the younger members of the clan would just as soon get rid of the allergic sufferer as to send away Fido or Pussy.

However, we cannot make light of this, for it is a very real emotional problem and a tough one for any shaman to tackle. It may suffice to build the pet his own castle by the back fence and banish him only as far as the yard; but sadly even that is often not enough, and it becomes a question of the pet or the allergic person's health.

The reader would be surprised at how often the pet comes first—especially between man and wife! And it is not difficult to imagine the resentment of other children in the family toward the one who has the asthma or eczema and who has robbed them of their dearly loved puppy or kitten. The allergic child suffers doubly—the loss of the pet and guilt that he is the cause of it all.

How does the wise shaman tackle such an emotional trauma?

Frankly, there is no good way that I know of. I try to soften the blow by telling the youngster involved that the pet has gone off to get married and to raise his (her) own family. Children can understand this aspect of pet life fairly well, and it provides their pet with a somewhat intriguing future. But even so, the trauma is such that unless allergy is severe, the benefits of such a step should be weighed carefully against the possible emotional damage. Before the pet is banished forever, it might be well to experiment a little to be sure animal danders are at fault in the matter. Banish Fido, for instance, only as far as the nearest kennel, a friend's house, out to Grandad's for a few weeks or months. Try things without him first, but be sure the house is cleaned of every trace of his presence as much as possible. Then, if the banishment *must* be final, do it gently. Take the children for a trip, and while they are gone, have the pet go off to a new home, preferably to some kind soul who will send back a picture of him being happy in his new life. Have some new interest available when the children return to divert them at least somewhat from their pain. Finally, there is always the possibility of substituting a nonallergenic animal.

"What's a nonallergenic animal?"

"Oh, some endearing snake or lizard."

"Oh now, Doctor! Brrrr!"

Well, yes, I can understand how such a substitution can play hobs with Mother's nervous system; but if she is a hardy soul and grits her teeth, it can work out pretty well. For example, several years ago I treated an animal-loving young fellow who, unhappily, suffered from multiple allergies. Tests showed that anything with fur or feathers was bound to make him worse. Rather light-heartedly I remarked, "What Jeff needs is a snake!" And then I forgot about it. Jeff's parents forgot about it. But Jeff didn't. In the end he didn't let them forget after all. Soon they were on the prowl for a snake, a harmless but attractive snake—if there is such a thing.

Attractive, I mean. They found just the snake, finally, a boa in a pet shop. They decided that it would be Jeff's Christmas present, but even the Asheville area can get chilly at that time of year. The pet store owner warned they would have to keep this tropical creature warm all the way back to their home some miles away. Fortunately for Jeff, his mother was one of the hardy ones. She wrapped the boa around her waist and kept him warm under her coat while Father drove. Jeff had his boa and diminished allergy symptoms, and everyone lived happily ever after. With a mother like that, how can Jeff help but make it!

Years ago I treated another animal lover who turned to an iguana when he had to give up the furred and feathered variety of pets. He brought this new addition to his family into the office on a leash one day and created predictable havoc among my waiting room patients and office staff.

Well, everyone or almost everyone likes animal stories—which is good; for in this world of considerable cruelty and aggression, the love of animals is a trait to be encouraged in children, because it teaches them kindness and compassion, gentleness and responsibility. It is a shame when a pet must go; and frequently it must, for the sake of the youngster's health. When it must, act with care, for there can be an emotional upheaval of first magnitude.

Incidentally, a pet isn't the only one to be blamed for providing allergens within the home other than those which naturally collect in such an environment (house dust, mold, and the like). Father can bring some pretty potent allergens home from work on his clothing and in his hair, a fact that is often overlooked by everyone, doctor included. For example, one man who worked in a soybean factory made his small son ill on a regular basis until it was discovered that the boy, sensitive to soybean, ran each evening to greet his returning daddy with a hug and a kiss. When the father changed clothes in the basement and showered before this nightly ritual, the boy's asthma diminished.

But the emotional climate within the family itself can aggravate and intensify the allergic individual's illness. The family arena can on occasion produce as much flat-out conflict as a boxing ring, with everyone coming out of his corner punching for real. Many a young writer, Asheville's own Thomas Wolfe included, has vividly depicted the love-hate duet so frequently carried on between man and wife, parent and child, sibling and sibling. Like many another institution, the family is stressed, often simply by the fact of its existence in a complex world. It is bombarded from without by a multitude of stimuli ranging from war and economic upheavals to occupational demands and conformity requirements. Such external pressures necessarily play a large role in family conflict, as individual members respond in varying ways to life changes and stresses. Thus, the father threatened by job insecurity or simply by boredom or lack of interest may respond with anxiety and depression. The mother, her horizons limited by child care and housework, may become irritable, dependent, and tense. Youngsters overstimulated by violence and the like, either on the TV screen or in the streets, may become aggressive and/or anxious. And each effect on one member will rebound among the others. The tentacles of stress reach around the family unit, which can no more exist in a vacuum than can you or I. We can see it happening on all sides. The father, anxious about his job, may turn upon the mother, whose self-esteem has already been sadly diminished by her narrowed world of small challenge. She, in turn, may take it out upon the children, who then war among themselves. The family is, as they say, the world in miniature.

As I sorted through the literature of allergy and emotions, the studies and observations made by practicing physicians and investigators in their laboratories, two emotions stood out as being strongly involved in the precipitation and aggravation of allergy, especially of asthma and eczema: anxiety and anger. Perhaps these powerful feelings are most universally damaging because they are apt to be prolonged. Grief can be savage and hurt to the core of our being; but maybe simply because it causes so much anguish, we slowly surmount it. Anger and anxiety can nibble away at our souls (as can guilt, I should add) year after year. We fear and we rage in childhood and old age. Only the tiniest infants seem immune to fear, although probably not to anger, as any mother knows who withholds bottle or breast a little too long.

Some of the things we are anxious about, death and pain, for instance, are real enough. Some of our anxieties, though, are of the die-a-thousand-deaths variety. We fear nebulous disaster, possible harm, a future threat. Such fears commonly have little utility and are maladaptions to actual stimuli or events. We could do without them. Unfortunately this is easier said than done. Anxiety may come to us as a legacy from early childhood. We may not even be aware that it exists or why; thus it is not easy to lay aside. It's like trying to gather up the fog to clear the highway ahead. The child constantly fearful of parental disapproval and rejection grows up as the anxious, dependent adult of low self-confidence and self-esteem. Often he will express such emotional disturbances in physical illness. Whether such emotional stress will lead to allergy or hypertension or peptic ulcer and the like will depend on other factors, perhaps genetic in the main. But parents must be aware that the emotional climate within the family may be as important to their child's future health as good nutrition, adequate sleep and exercise, trips to the dentist every six months, and a yearly physical at the family doctor's. We know, for instance, that malnutrition at certain critical stages of human development can actually diminish intelligence as well as bodily structure. Unhappily, I do not believe that we are as keenly aware that deprivation of affection, of love, can be as critical.

There is, of course, no way to protect a child against all anxiety, all anger, or any other emotion such as grief and guilt. Even if there were, it would not necessarily be a good thing. Adversity is a part of our training for life. And to be emotionally becalmed would be a great bore. But we can diminish powerful emotional stress by loving our children; by communicating that love clearly; and by supporting and encouraging them to overcome difficulties, to develop as strong, confident, and loving persons.

A mother knows that when the crawling baby stands up to toddle, he is in for bumps and bruises. She cannot prevent this unless she follows him about constantly, hangs on to his suspenders or the like, and continually shouts, "Watch out!"–"Don't touch!"–"Be careful!" If she does do this, she will chain him to the floor with fears. Of course, there are dangers that she must foresee and forestall, such as those of hot stoves and steep staircases, but in general she must let him take his licks and learn by them how to toddle successfully so that he may walk with confidence later. She must teach the need for caution without instilling fear. And when the fall comes, as it must, she should encourage him to rise again and toddle on. The whole spectrum of our lives is mirrored by that toddler crossing the room. We must not fear so much that we do not dare; and when we fall, we must rise again. If parents wish to see their children mature to healthy, happy, productive adulthood, they must ensure that the family supports, encourages, and allows the development of independence in its emerging stages. It is impossible to erase all conflict, all emotional stress, but parents must remember that the child who is chained by overprotection, robbed of self-esteem by rejection, scolded more often than comforted, is often the child who sits and howls at fate. And that howl may well be expressed in such physical illness as chronic allergy made far worse than it need be.

Now let us reduce these somewhat general statements to some specifics.

We noted earlier that it is very important when a child is having an asthma attack not to show fear, that your fear can intensify his symptoms. When parents hit the panic button during such a crisis, they intensify the child's anxiety, and his fear is already considerable. Such intensification can be serious indeed, even fatal. But even when the child is not actually suffering asthma symptoms, if parents reinforce residual anxiety by exhorting him continually not to attempt this, not to overexert, not to do that lest it bring on an asthma attack, it is quite understandable that the child will not only suffer continual anxiety, but his development will be retarded, even distorted. Such a child can become emotionally crippled, can even withdraw from life's challenges so completely as to become psychopathic.

In her discussion with me, Debora Phillips presented a somewhat unique way of estimating such fears and a technique by which the child can communicate his anxiety to his parents so that both he and they can remain in control of fear:

> A child can learn to use a subjective anxiety scale–this scale goes from 0 to 100, and he can be taught that 0 is when you feel totally free of any nervousness, any tension, any anxiety, while 100 is like the panic button; it's the most anxiety he could possible experience. He can learn to use this scale as a cue to himself so that he learns when his anxiety starts going up and he can perhaps tell his parents when it gets to, say, 20 without waiting until it gets as high as 90. This is a kind of warning system than can be set up between parents and the asthmatic child, and then between parents and the doctor. This child has to learn to be subjective–that 50 is halfway to 100–so that's quite a bit of anxiety. 30 is kind of butterfly feelings; it's quite a bit of nervousness but it's not panic, it's not extreme tension.

Worthwhile as the above regime is in controlling anxiety for both parents and child, it has the added value of teaching the child responsibility for his own illness. This is a giant step toward maturity. And maturity for the allergic child is another specific for parents to zoom in on. Investigators have demonstrated that fostering independence in allergic children can diminish the effects of their chronic symptoms. Thus, frustration of the natural urges toward maturity and self-sufficiency through overprotection may actually increase the severity of the child's illness. Parents are very naturally going to wish to protect their severely allergic child from recurrent bouts with his illness if they can, but they must learn to walk a thin line here to keep from overprotecting and frustrating him. It is not easy. One of the ways to do this is to begin by giving him some responsibility for the avoidance measures necessary to control his allergy and even in the matter of the medications he may need to take. He must also learn, even if he has to do it the hard way, what limitations, if any, his allergy imposes—overexertion, for instance; or chilling; or overeating and the like. Or if he is allergic to chocolate but is downed by temptation, then the lesson must be his to learn.

It is surprising how often in families where conflict exists before allergy, the allergic child serves as a sort of fulcrum for an emotional conflict. The mother, for instance, may become overinvolved with the allergic child to the exclusion of other real problems. She may find his illness a way to avoid solution of emotional conflicts arising between herself and her husband. Studies of families of patients suffering persistent and severe allergy indicate a somewhat characteristic pattern. Such families appear to be rigid and overintrusive. There is little privacy within the family circle and much overprotectiveness. Such families seem to create barriers to outside social contact and act sufficient unto themselves. And when one of their members becomes ill, they appear to use his illness as a protection from their own conflicts. It is not hard to understand, then, how a child who has developed asthma from the combined action of an infection and an allergen can have his symptoms reinforced in such a family until he arrives at the point where he responds with asthma to any emotional stress.

This problem of overprotection is a tricky one. We can exhort parents, particularly mothers, not to overprotect, but when does protection become overprotection? It is natural and wholly desirable that parents protect their children. And when a child is ill, especially severely so, then parents must protect him far more than they normally would. Perhaps if we can be sensitive to signs of frustration in the child–temper tantrums, stubbornness, and the like–we can recognize when we have stepped over the line from healthy protection to overprotection. It is something parents must be alert for, certainly.

This discussion leads us to the value of developing self-confidence in the child and a satisfactory self-image, both of which are vital to a healthy emotional and physical adulthood. How does one do this? Encourage! Support! Praise when praise is due. This should be as true for the normal, healthy child as for the allergic one. It makes no sense to limit a child's physical or mental development or pride of accomplishment unnecessarily. When limits of one kind or another must be set because of physical (or mental, for that matter) handicaps, then parents should cast about for substitutes that such a child can turn to for pleasure and pride and accomplishment. The self-confidence of the adult is born in the child. To function, child and man must know that he "can do." For instance, in a study of children with eczema, it was found that the majority of them were withdrawn and anxious and beset by feelings of insecurity. They were typically dependent youngsters and felt programmed for failure. A minority of the group studied overcompensated for their lack of self-confidence by being aggressive and given to temper tantrums. Either of these two characteristics can be carried into adulthood.

So, again, what does make sense is positive reinforcement of the traits we wish to see our children develop and carry out into the world. Parents of allergic children, and for that matter parents of children who suffer any chronic illness, must refrain from negative reinforcement. Illness should not have utility or be an escape from responsibility. Parents must not allow the ill child to set himself up as a little dictator–which he will do, given half the chance! Not only is such negative reinforcement generally unfair to the rest of the family, but it provides the ill child with a distorted view of life. And it can cripple the future adult. Once he has gone out from the family castle, few people will answer his beck and call or be overwhelmed by his continuing disabilities. So there is no need for parents to be led down such a primrose path by the imaginative ploys of their allergic youngster. They must have the courage to discipline him as they would a nonallergic child, to expect from him the same sort of behavior.

Let us return to Ms. Phillips, who says of such allergic children:

> That is not to say that he should not get a lot of positive reinforcement as we would recommend for any child. For starters, when there is a lot of negative interaction between parents and children, I recommend that parents begin to compliment their children four times a day or something very minimal. This is a concrete thing that parents can do—they should keep a record of it, checking off four times a day when they've given a compliment. [I hasten to add to Ms. Phillips advice—don't ever let the youngster find that checkoff slip!] The compliment should be about something they can point out to the child that he has done; not "You're great" or "You're terrific," but "You did a really good job with that" or "That's a nice problem you solved on that paper—you did well on that" or "You look really neat the way you're wearing your shirt today." Something that the child can accept, that is genuine and true. Parents should not lie about this but they should, whenever it's humanly possible, give the child positive reinforcement through compliments and praise. This is especially helpful for the child who does not think well of himself, and we know that many children, whether they have learning disabilities or allergies, are children who fall into this category because of their difficulty. Along with positive reinforcement, if the parent can be helped to refrain from making any negative or downgrading remarks about the child, especially in front of the child, it would be very helpful to his self-image, for his feelings of normalcy and adequacy as a human being and as a child. If the same situation always or consistently seems to trigger an allergic reaction, it would be well to look closely at the situation to see if it has negative emotional elements within it.

I second the motion! More than that, I believe there would be a lot less emotional ill health about if the idea of positive reinforcement were carried over into a good part of adult life. A great many people need desperately to be complimented and praised. Husbands should go out of their way to praise housebound wives, remembering that their bosses and fellow workers praise them (or should) for their jobs well done! If the husband does not praise the housewife, who will? The children could care less that the wash is whiter than white and that the bathroom sparkles, although they might get off an occasional "Hey, Mom, this stuff tastes neat!" A person needs a bit more than that. She needs to be told sometimes that her job is important, too, and that it is thoroughly appreciated on an adult level. I think this feeling of being unappreciated for one's life work of motherhood and housewifery lies behind a good deal of the thrust of the women's liberation movement. We have downgraded the raising of the future generation until we appear to feel that it is a job for the incompetent, the unskilled, and least intelligent.

An employer, if he is wise and wishes to get the best from his employees, will be as lavish with his praise as he is with his raise.

Accentuate the positive! Refrain from putting down! These are two cardinal rules for keeping everyone happy.

In varying ways and to varying degrees the allergic member of the family can contribute to conflict within the home. If his allergy is chronic and moderate to severe, it can impose limitations on other members' activities. This often gives rise to resentment, as we have noted in our discussion of the problem of pets. Another example would be an asthmatic wife and a smoking husband; they present a clear conflict of interest—her health and his habit. Believe it or not, it can end in divorce court. Even if he gives up smoking (and I have known husbands who would not) or goes out in the garage to satisfy his need for nicotine, the chances are good that he will resent it bitterly. He may even be convinced that her asthma is a put-on, a way to get him to give up the weed, or, worse still, to punish him or get back at him or spite him. On her side, she may well be angered by his sad moans and interpret them as begrudging her her health. She may begin to wonder if he doesn't prefer his tobacco to her. Nonsmokers can get pretty belligerent about the fouling of the air they have to breathe as it is. You may not believe it, but I had a smoking mother resent the instruction that she cease smoking in the child's vicinity because it was making him ill! We humans have odd values on occasion!

The allergic-to-food member who must follow a somewhat rigid diet to stay symptom-free can find himself considered a drag by the rest of the family, especially by Mother. Either she must prepare two separate menus for every meal, or the nonallergic persons must learn to tolerate some of the patient's limited diet items. Rather naturally, unless neatly handled, this state of affairs can generate a good bit of resentment and hostility. It is no easy matter to arrange such menus that will fit the mother's budget, time, and energy yet meet the needs and demands of everyone. She may also have to contend with the allergic child's feeling that he is being punished by not being able to eat what his siblings are served. This can be especially true of younger children who do not fully understand their problem. Mother will have to be unusually creative in her cooking and diplomatic in her dealings.

Mother will also have to contend with a good bit of anxiety. A child who is severely allergic to bee or wasp venom can be the vortex of a thousand fears until he is safely desensitized. Equally, a child exceedingly hypersensitive to food, especially when very young, can be the source of constant worry. Mother will fear that he may be served up some goody by a well-meaning neighbor or by one of his friends. Worse still, she may be anxious that she herself might contribute to his illness in a forgetful moment by putting some forbidden food into her cooking. For instance, a child can be so exceedingly allergic to eggs that even a very small portion can make him extremely ill. Yet eggs are hard to avoid. They are in many a prepackaged food, and recipes call for them in abundance. It is easy to slip up on this kind of thing. And if she does, her feelings of guilt are also easy to comprehend. If Father adds his criticism to the child's symptoms, Mother can be thoroughly devastated.

The allergic family member who must avoid certain pollens at certain times of year or places that breed mold in excess may dictate where and when a family spends its vacations or how family outings are planned. Again we have the ingredients for resentment–and blame. "Aw, why can't we go camping like we used to? Just because dumb old Jimmy starts to sneeze! Boy!"

And there is nothing to match the furor when a favorite, long-awaited outing has to be canceled because the allergic family member has broken out with hives or begun to wheeze.

It is not easy for parents to cope with the problems of a chronically ill child. Unconsciously, they may resent the drain severe allergy can make on the family finances, while siblings watch bitterly as the allergic child's room is refurbished with new nonallergenic items and toys. Parents can grow weary of constant explaining, first to the allergic child as to why his beloved old stuffed teddy bear has to head for the garbage can, then to the brothers and sisters as to why the teddy has to be replaced by bright and shiny plastic toys. This constant walking of a tightrope so as not to give the impression of favoring the allergic child over his siblings can be exhausting. There is enough rivalry within a family without this.

Sometimes this sort of stress is such that it sets one parent against the other. Harassed, the mother may blame the child's allergy on the father's family because there is a history of allergy there and obviously it is his genes that brought them all this trouble. He may retaliate that she coddles and pampers the child too much, that she is spoiling him rotten. The accused parent, and it seems to be most often the mother, complicates an already unhealthy situation by assuming a considerable burden of guilt for the child's illness. And such conflict between parents can only damage a child already made emotionally vulnerable by chronic illness.

One of the most devastating things a family can do is to treat the allergic sufferer in their midst as a malingerer or hypochondriac or neurotic. Given the sometimes diffuse symptoms of nervous system or gastrointestinal allergy, this is a frequent response. Parents or spouses are apt to grow impatient with the allergic victim's general feelings of unwellness and fatigue. They, in their good health, may also become a shade contemptuous. This can damage the already poor self-image of the ill member and decrease his self-confidence, what there is of it.

Finally, parents are often afraid to discipline the allergic child in a normal manner for fear of setting him off. In this situation, the child quickly learns to use his illness as a club. He finds he can manipulate the family to suit his own needs, and he does. We noted this trap earlier in the book, and I am aware that it is easy to say "Discipline as you would any other child," and difficult to do it when your child suddenly has a severe asthma attack following such discipline. Yet, if parents can keep in mind the great harm they can do by allowing the child to use his allergy as a crutch, it may be easier. Reinforcing illness can only make illness more prolonged and maladaption more deeply engraved.

17

Coping with the Cold, Cruel World

A spinning potter's wheel whirls us ceaselessly through life and we are thumped and fingered in and out of shape even though we retain a recognizable form—a bowl, a vase, a pitcher. The events of our early childhood set the rough outlines of that form; but the great world outside, beginning with the family and ending with our society, adds, discards, and shapes the ornamental additional structures of our lives—re-forms a handle, changes a rim, curves a new base. We are not quite the same person from year to year, yet we retain the self of our genetic inheritance, our beginning years, and our individuality.

As we have seen, the family begins the job once we are plopped down upon the potter's wheel as a somewhat formless shape, a hunk of malleable clay. The makeup of the clay itself has quite a bit to do with the finished product. It may determine whether the wheel will turn out a utilitarian bowl or an ornamental vase, for we are not all born alike. As we have noted, almost all of us have some little imperfection of one kind or another, and some of us more so than others. Most of us, too, arrive on the wheel with some special gift the world needs desperately, so let us hope that the potter does not smooth it to oblivion. Now, having exhausted both clay and wheel, I'll get down to specifics.

How can the chronically allergic child be equipped and how should he be equipped to be able to move out into the world under his own power?

Maturity, self-confidence, self-esteem are his best weapons for coping with the cold, cruel world. As we have seen, parents can provide him with these weapons by giving him love, support, and encouragement, and by allowing him to develop his independence. Unfortunately, parents don't come equipped with instinctive knowledge about all possible situations. They are inclined to grope for answers even as the child gropes his way to manhood. Mistakes are made, but then to err is human—which accounts for the many books on child raising and how to be a parent.

The first and very natural step parents should take when they suspect the child is ill is to consult a physician. If he believes the problem is allergy and refers the child to an allergist, parents should be so guided. Allergy treated early in the game has a far greater chance of being mild, even though sensitivity to allergens may never wholly disappear. Such allergy can be controlled by proper management measures and/or prophylactic drugs so that it can be little more than one of life's minor nuisances. Even individuals who suffered severe asthma during childhood have gone on into the world of professional sports and college teams successfully. Some have even made it in the armed services with little or no trouble. Obviously, nobody ever told these youngsters that they were handicapped! It must be said, however, that allergic individuals, especially those suffering moderate-to-severe asthma and eczema, tend to choose less rigorous careers, and often as a matter of necessity.

These two allergic illnesses, asthma and eczema, when severe and intractable, can be real tragedies for their victims. They can cripple! I cannot emphasize strongly enough the importance of early attention to allergy. And parents must keep in mind that hay fever, rhinitis, and gastrointestinal allergy can progress to asthma. Early management measures of avoidance of allergens and perhaps medication often as not can prevent this sad progression.

Once the fact of allergy is established and the child is under an allergist's care, the parents then must avoid a number of pitfalls that can thwart the child's natural development as he moves out into the world. Nor are parents alone in this responsibility. Teachers especially have a vital role to play, for the school becomes the world in miniature for youngsters as they move one heady step from home. Most of us can remember at least one teacher who turned us on and made a great difference in our lives. Alas, most of us also can remember at least one teacher who turned us all the way off!

School for the chronically ill child can be a difficult business at best, a nightmare at worst. He is likely to miss many classroom hours because of his illness, while his schoolwork may suffer because he often operates at less than peak capacity. The teacher of such a child must be even more patient, more understanding than usual, yet must avoid giving the appearance of favoritism. He will do the child no favors if he makes it seem that the child is "teacher's pet." Favoritism is grossly unfair in the classroom and deadly to the will-to-learn as well as to young self-images. Children quickly sense such injustice and are apt to turn cruelly on the "pet."

The teacher can, however, take extra time to see that the allergic youngster keeps abreast of his classmates. Perhaps he can work something out with the parents or suggest a tutor temporarily or even arrange to visit the child's home to help him stay up with his work. He should be aware that it is vitally important for the chronically ill child to feel adequate, to feel that he can cope. He should not be allowed to fall behind. I do not know whether teachers receive information about common childhood illness during their training, but perhaps they should, at least insofar as a child's behavior may stem from illness. If they were taught to recognize and handle such behavior properly, a good bit of childhood's trauma might be avoided. Certainly the chances are good that the chronically ill child who is treated as the classroom dunce is not going to make a very satisfactory adjustment in later life.

There are several specific things a teacher can do to safeguard the allergic child's health during school hours. Since an allergic child is so often sensitive to temperature changes, he should not sit by an open window. Nor should he shower after gym and then go out in the cold. Because dust is often a factor, he should not clean erasers and the like. Nor should he be exposed to strong fumes, especially if he suffers from asthma or rhinitis. And since it is often important that an allergic child, especially an asthmatic child, feel secure, parents and teacher should get together on the possible need for medication during the school day. Perhaps the teacher could keep the child's medicine in her desk, with the child made aware that it was available. Frequently, medication taken at the first sign of a wheeze can abort an asthma attack. In this vein, if teachers were instructed in the fundamentals and symptoms of allergy during their training, they might be able to recognize the allergic child in their classroom and suggest to parents that he be seen by a doctor. Such a step could save some parents a great deal of misunderstanding and some children a great deal of grief.

Teachers also should be careful not to scold or make snide remarks about the child who constantly sniffles, sneezes, or coughs, no matter how disruptive he is. "Stop sniffling!" is not only an intensely embarrassing and mortifying command but an all-but-impossible one for the allergic child to obey. Perhaps the teacher could ask privately for an explanation or consult the parents or send the child to the school nurse. The worst thing she could do is call him down publicly for something he cannot help. Considering that he is probably already considerably embarrassed and distressed by the disruption he is making, as little attention as possible should be drawn to him. Even if he *were* deliberately disrupting the class, I should think additional attention would be what he was hoping for.

In general, I think it can be said that the allergic child who is receiving proper treatment for his allergy and proper support and encouragement from his parents will miss very little school and will easily be able to stay up with his peers. It is commonly the youngster whose allergy is either unrecognized or not adequately controlled who will present the greatest problem for the teacher. She must then walk a tightrope even as parents often do. She must help the child as much as she can, but without singling him out as "special" or making him feel "different." She must make him feel secure in the classroom without smothering him. She must support his self-image and sense of adequacy, yet not overtax him. But let us not overburden our already overloaded teacher. She must not develop guilt and a sense of failure because of temporary lapses in both the physical and the emotional health of the allergic child! In the main, if she is aware of his problem and has the good of her students at heart, she will do right by him as she does right by the other, perhaps more fortunate youngsters in her classroom.

We must go back to Mother here, though, for she plays the major role in helping her child step out of the home into the world via the school. One of the specific things she can do is to refrain from making her allergic child appear "different" to his peers, for this can be the kiss of death. For instance, she should consider that either riding the schoolbus or walking to school, as the other youngsters do, is healthy until proved otherwise. If she insists on driving her child to and from school while all his friends ride the bus or walk, she is setting him apart as clearly as if she tied a label to him or put a ribbon in his hair. There may be wet, chill mornings when his health dictates such a move; but when the weather is good, she should put the brakes on her inclination to protect and imagine instead the singsong voices, "Hoo, boy, Johnny's gotta ride to school with his momma!"

I think, too, that the mother and the doctor ought to get their heads together to help the teacher by providing her with some detailed instructions. Perhaps the allergist could write a brief note for the mother to give her child's teacher. It could summarize the child's allergy and the things he must avoid at school in order to stay well. Here, for example, could be a sample Note To Teacher:

> John Doe has severe asthma that is due to inhalants and foods and which is aggravated by temperature changes. Ragweed and dust are the chief inhalant allergens he must avoid. He is presently taking desensitization shots for these, but he has not yet built up to a tolerance level. If he is exposed to too much of either of these inhalants, he may start wheezing.
>
> The ragweed pollen is in the air from about the middle of August until frost; therefore, during this time, at least for this year, it would be better for him not to play football, baseball, and the like outdoors.
>
> As far as dust exposure goes, for this year he should not be asked to clean erasers, stack old books, sweep, or tumble or play on dusty floor mats.
>
> The chief foods that cause his allergy are milk and chocolate. So as not to make it more noticeable to the other children, I have instructed his mother to use a milk substitute (soybean) which he will bring to school either in a thermos or unused small milk container. He has been instructed to eat no chocolate.
>
> His medication for asthma is a blue pill, and his mother will supply you with some. They are very effective if given as directed at the slightest hint of wheezing. The child is instructed to tell you immediately when this occurs. The pill may be repeated every four hours if needed. If the boy's asthma becomes worse, call his mother and she will take him to the doctor.
>
> It is all right for him to take gym classes unless (1) it causes him to wheeze and (2) he does have to go outdoors after exercise or right after taking a shower.
>
> I am hoping that with careful allergic management most or all of these restrictions will be removed.

Teachers and parents perhaps should also get together so that unrealistic goals are not set for the allergic child. Pressure to succeed can cause considerable anxiety for the child and can only aggravate his allergy. This includes physical activities as well as mental, for we must remember that allergic children often suffer from fatigue, and their sleep may be disturbed by asthma or eczema.

School sports can pose a real and possibly traumatic problem for the severely allergic child, especially for a boy. Physical education teachers of both sexes sometimes seem to lose sight of the individual youngsters in their pursuit of physical perfection. For some reason, they appear suspicious of parents and their little scrawled "excuse" notes—perhaps with good reason. Many parents seem to try to overprotect in this area especially, to mitigate with an "excuse" the hurt which seems so often to arise in this part of the school day. A good deal of valid criticism has been leveled at school physical education programs because they tend to establish a school elite from which the majority of youngsters are barred. In many schools the gym and playing fields are hogged by this elite to the detriment of the rest of the students. Team sports have their place, I suppose, but I think the current overemphasis has gone a long way in developing the great American spectator rather than physically fit persons who can carry their exercise and fun and games all the way to old age.

The allergic child has special problems in the school gym and out on the playing fields. Dusty exercise mats, overexertion, overheating, showers and then having to go out in the cold—all are possible triggers for allergy, as we have seen. Thus, some of the physical education program may be off limits for the moderately to severely allergic. It can, however, be very hard on a youngster's self-image and self-confidence to be left sitting on the sidelines, excuse clutched in his hand, his image of weakling, of physically unfit, of sissy projected not only to his peers but to himself. To avoid such emotional damage, and to benefit the child physically, I believe that time and thought should be given to arranging substitutes for such children. It is vital that allergic children, or children suffering other types of chronic illness, be encouraged and aided in excelling in some physical endeavor that is within their limitations. I also have a sneaking suspicion that they will be the fortunate ones in the end who can continue their sports—tennis, golf, swimming, or whatever—all the way down to their doddering years, whereas the team players of the elite squads all too often will become overweight spectators comfortable in their overstuffed chairs in front of the TV game-of-the week.

Physical exertion is valuable on two fronts. It not only benefits the body, but it also benefits the mind. It helps ease emotional stress, particularly anxiety and depression. A proper program in the schools should go out of its way to build, rather than tear down, the self-confidence of *all* children. With this goal in mind, it must be tailored to individual differences of growth rate, muscular development, physical defects, and the like. The allergic child is not the only one forced into the role of perpetual bystander by the overemphasis on teams and winning. Alternatives to competitive sports, however, must not be just another class for physical "incompetents." Such a program must work at the goal of building self-confidence, physical health and skill, pride in self, and pleasure in exerting one's body. It must teach a vital lesson to last a lifetime, that games can be played simply for the fun of it, that exertion practiced simply because it makes the body and mind feel good is an excellent way of life.

I truly believe that physical education programs in many schools have failed to train American children in the necessity and pleasure of continuing regular exercise in adult life, not only as an adjunct to bodily health but as a means of countering emotional stress. Since few of us are fortunate enough not to have some physical or mental imperfection that imposes some limiting factor on life's possibilities, I do not believe in "excuses." I do not think even severely limited youngsters should learn to sit upon the sidelines to watch others have all the fun and receive all the accolades. I am sure that this can be nothing if not devastating to their egos. Therefore, I believe parents should make a special effort to work out some way to compensate in this part of their children's education. I also believe that schools which have the good of their students at heart will do their very best to equalize nonmaterial rewards for young people, to spread recognition and pride over a wide variety of endeavors, lest we put down so many that they give up trying or turn to less socially rewarding pursuits–purse snatching, for instance.

And just to prove my point, I have treated youngsters for severe asthma who, in later years, have sent me clippings to show that they played college football, made the first team in basketball, and the like. Several of my ex-patients have been star college players! Physical and emotional crippling because of allergy is not necessary. All children, allergic and nonallergic alike, need positive reinforcement for their self-image, self-esteem, self-confidence. It should be the number one priority of the schools, even as it should be within the family.

Adolescents, young adults who are only one step away from the cold, cruel world, especially need encouragement, and their self-confidence and self-image supported. While they are struggling mightily to free themselves from the parental shadow, they are also pretty anxious about their ability to cope with the real world beyond the safety of the family circle. I am not sure that as a society we have done much to help them achieve independence or offered much in the way of positive reinforcement. Many young people have difficulty finding jobs when they leave high school, and this is a powerful negative reinforcement to their self-esteem and self-confidence. Many who go on to higher education find themselves lost in huge multi-universities, where those most uncertain or most limited by physical or emotional difficulties have little chance of finding help—or of help finding them. The young adult is primed to receive the wisdom and understanding of adults who stand outside the family circle at this stage of development, yet there appears to be less chance than ever before for them to have such nonfamily guidance—unless they foul up; unless they unhappily come to the attention of guidance counselors or authorities of one sort or another. The young, especially when they are moving out of the family castle and beyond the moat, need a sense of identity, a model to emulate, a wise old hand to provide ideas and possibilities, new ways of thinking, and help in evaluating their goals.

It is a critical time of life. And the young adult who suffers from moderate-to-severe allergy may have several extraordinary strikes against him—hormonal alterations that may trigger and aggravate his symptoms, and emotional stress in the form of anxiety, especially, which may do the same thing. It is a cruel blow of fate to have to make the giant step out into the world eczematous or asthmatic or burdened by other allergy symptoms. Such a blow may turn some youngsters back into the family fold, especially if their independence has already been stifled, their self-confidence crippled.

Young adults, and older ones also, often come a cropper over the social graces. We humans are creatures of custom, and for some reason or other the social niceties assume great importance in our relationships with each other—perhaps because they simply oil the social wheels, smooth down the rough places, make the whole move quietly and with ease. In any case our social life plays a large role in our sense of well-being, our feelings of adequacy and self-esteem. When we are, or at least feel that we are, attractive to others, can get along well with them, can offer meaningful input into our contacts with them, we are usually quite happy with our lot. Conversely, we can be emotionally shattered by social goofs, feelings of being unattractive to others, of being unwanted among our fellows, and the like. The man-without-a-country syndrome is pretty devastating, for a good part of our self-image is derived from the sort of echoes we bounce off our own kind. We fear being judged by our fellows, and thus to a certain extent we fear each other.

Because allergy is not very well understood, even among doctors, allergic persons often feel such judgment harshly. The victim of somewhat severe skin allergy may find revulsion or simply imagine it in the glances of others and become thoroughly depressed. The victim of the constant sniffle and sneeze of rhinitis or the wheeze and disability of asthma may believe others view him with contempt. Smooth traffic with one's kind is difficult when one's face and hands and other visible surfaces are disfigured, or when one must drop out of gatherings or activities because of respiratory difficulties. It is not necessarily the situation itself that causes the emotional distress, but rather how the individual perceives it. The strong, self-confident ego can take such things in stride ordinarily; but those of lowly self-esteem are often badly hurt, emotionally and physically, for that hurt can as easily be reflected in increased severity of their allergic symptoms as it can in anxiety and depression.

How the allergy sufferer reacts to such situations has its roots back in early childhood and some of its branches in his later life experiences in the family, in school, and out in the world. He may have much to be grateful to his parents for, or much to condemn. If his parents loved him well but did not overprotect, if they encouraged him to independence and to be responsible, if they gave him the inner strength that comes with a satisfactory self-image, then he will be able to keep the faith that his allergy will improve and that if others look askance at his symptoms, it is a measure of their own weakness, not of his. Because he is mature he will have the self-discipline to follow doctor's orders. He will understand that fear and anxiety only make matters worse. He will not bemoan his fate and take out his self-pity in hostility toward others. Nor will he retire to some inner cave to cower, nor return to the bosom of his family. No, this is the fellow who will sally forth into the world and put as good a face (or what's left of it) on matters as possible.

If food or drink are the allergenic substances responsible for an individual's symptoms, he may encounter some embarrassing if superficial social problems. Let us say, for instance, that he has just received an invitation to an elegant formal banquet which he would very much like to attend for business and/or social reasons. (There is a bit of the climber in us all!) However, cruel experience has taught him that there are allergens in affairs like this just waiting to ambush him. Unhappily, he is allergic to both eggs and wheat, which, of course, are found in almost everything. Even more unhappily, he reacts to them with hives and angioedema. In fact, his face blows up like a balloon within minutes of ingesting even a tiny bit of egg and only a little less slowly after eating wheat. So there he roosts, uncomfortably upon the horns of a dilemma. Should he accept? Or refuse and risk losing out on various things of value to him? If he accepts, should he eat everything put before him, knowing pretty well what would happen? Or should he try to pick and choose among the various dishes and risk mortally offending his hostess?

Well, any wise shaman would advise him to do none of these. He should simply pick up the phone and matter-of-factly explain his problem to his hostess. After all, he cannot help being allergic, can he? Anyway, the chances are excellent that she will not only understand his predicament but will proudly prepare him some sort of eggless, wheatless concoction and slip it to him.

It's really a matter of common sense, isn't it?

It is even simpler for the mother of an allergic child invited to a party. She can not only call up ahead of time to explain the situation but can even carry over a bit of the child's nonallergic fare. Giving a party is even simpler, for if it can be arranged buffet style; the allergic person, whether child or adult, can inconspicuously pick and choose among a number of items. With a little foresight and effort the social aspects of food allergy can be managed with a minimum of difficulty. Even realistic Shirley Temple–type cocktails or tomato juice mimicking a Bloody Mary can forestall the kind of jovial joshing the nonalcoholic or the allergic-to-liquor individuals so often get.

The respiratory sensitivity of some asthmatic and rhinitis sufferers makes the choice of a number of occupations off-limits, notably those in which there is exposure to strong odors, fumes, smoke, dust, and the like. Bakers, for instance, can develop asthma or rhinitis from their constant contact with flour. Such limitations, I suppose, might have emotional impact on the allergic person, but since the world is wide and full of a number of vocations, my guess is that the impact would be neither great nor lasting. In the same manner persons with sensitive skin might not be able to handle strong chemicals or even certain materials such as silk or fur; but, again, except perhaps if the allergy developed after one was well established in a trade, emotional stress should not be too great. It may be simply a matter of trimming one's occupational sails but not having to reef them. Of course if it is a matter of a job loss, period, or of a loss of self-esteem in some manner, then the allergic individual may develop undue anxiety or hostility, with all that that may mean for his allergy.

In other ways, however, occupations, like the schools, can be the cause of considerable emotional stress, which may add an additional load to the allergic individual's precarious balance. Boredom in one's daily work, alienation from or indifference to one's job accomplishments, hostility toward one's superiors or fellow workers—all these can cause powerful emotional stresses. A further stress factor, nonallergenic in character, is that imposed by the noise generated in many occupations. Recent studies have shown a surprising correlation between noise intensity and ill health, both physical and mental. We also know that some individuals have difficulty becoming habituated to noise and are far more susceptible to its harmful effects than other persons. Noise can actually set up the conditions of emotional stress by the release of catecholamines.

Other types of pollution of the environment in and out of the individual's occupation can cause emotional stress for the allergic and the nonallergic individual alike. Strong fumes and odors not only precipitate allergy directly by their inflammatory action on organ tissues, but they may also generate enough anger and disgust to lower the allergic individual's tolerance level. Anxiety about the air one breathes when it is so fouled as to make breathing difficult may be almost as much of a component in the asthma attacks of victims of pollution as the polluting substances themselves. Certainly the incidence of asthma rises dramatically during pollution episodes.

All in all, our jobs, the environment in which we live, the way we are educated, our relationships with each other—all influence in one way or another our emotional and physical health. Like fish, we swim in a sea of social factors. They can support us well or strand us on a beach to wither and die. But it is up to us in the end to learn how to best stay in the water and survive.

18

How a Shaman Lays It On!

I spoke wistfully a few chapters back of how simple it would be to load the emotional problems of my allergic patients on little ships and launch them toward the distant sea. I would be just as pleased if I could shake my gourd rattle three times, intone a proper incantation, and escort my radiant, symptom-free patients out my office door.

Naturally, since neither of these pleasant prospects is possible, I must then work at my trade. And I must begin the moment a patient seats himself for the first time across the desk from me and turns an expectant face in my direction. He came to me to be cured, and I must see to it that he is.

First, of course, I must find out what ails him. By this, I do not mean simply what his symptoms are. That would be easy enough. He would just have to rattle off a list, a sort of shopping list of assorted aches and pains and discomforts. Unfortunately for both of us, matters are likely to be far more complex than this. Well, we shall see.

As we have already noted, the patient's history is the first step and a vital one. How the wise shaman conducts this initial contact with his patient is exceedingly important. Hopefully, he will be able to establish a therapeutic relationship quickly, a relationship that will help effect a "cure." It is a major feature of treatment, and we shamans should never be too pushed, too busy to give it our full attention. It can make all the difference.

Ordinarily, most of my patients are referred by their family doctors. The very fact of referral often gives such patients the feeling that theirs is an unusual illness. They arrive in my office believing that at last their symptoms, which have continued in spite of prior treatment, will be alleviated. They tend to feel that they are now in the hands of an expert. This is a giant plus for my side. Faith in one's doctor and hope for a cure are all-important. It is up to me to hang on to this advantage, and I do. Grimly. It is that highly prized ingredient—the power of suggestion.

As we have noted, the initial interview begins prosaically enough; but while my questions sound simple, there actually is an art to taking a patient's history. Even though information is what he seeks, the shaman tries also to convey the idea that he is interested in the patient's troubles, that he cares. However, he would be wise to start off with a general approach before tackling the specifics. For instance, as soon as his patient appears comfortably seated over there across the desk, he might ask, "Dr. X tells me you are having difficulties. Tell me about your problem . . . ."

It is amazing how much a doctor can divine about his patient from the latter's answer to this one broad question. Some patients will simply go down the shopping list of symptoms. Others will exaggerate their symptoms, while still others will do the opposite and make light of their troubles. Most will answer in such a way that the shaman can discover what is most important about his illness to the patient and how he regards it—in a word, his emotional overlay, his emotional set.

Even the type of relationship that will exist, at least initially, between shaman and patient may be revealed in this broad response. In a way the choice of one of these three types—the active-passive relationship, the guidance-cooperation type, or the adult-to-adult model—is tacitly the patient's, although some doctors operate solely along one set of guidelines in this matter. In the active-passive relationship, the patient becomes as a little child and the doctor assumes a parent's role. In the guidance-cooperation relationship, the patient follows doctor's orders, recognizing him as an authority and cooperating with him on this basis. The adult-to-adult relationship is one most usually met in the treatment of long-term, chronic illness. In this relationship the patient does not defer so completely to the doctor's authority as in the other two types, and he takes far more responsibility for his own treatment. All three types, or modifications of them, will often operate during the treatment of a single patient. In long-term allergy treatment the last will probably be the most pervasive.

So, we have begun with the general question and set the initial relationship with our patient. We have then gone on to get the specifics of birthdate, past problems, childhood illnesses, and the like. What next?

Every doctor, I should suppose, has his own way of doing things. And I have mine. Right about here I would probably have my patient tell me about his allergy in his own words, although I would no doubt have to interject a few specific or general questions now and again. For instance, when he tells me about his symptoms, say, his wheezing, I would want to know when he has such attacks, where, and what might have preceded them. On a more general level, I would like to know about his diet, his sleep pattern, and his feelings. I would ask questions about his occupation and his home, not only to try to track down allergens present in his environment but to also try to discover if emotional stresses might be involved—conflict with a boss, for instance; or dissatisfaction with his home neighborhood. Very naturally, I would try to elicit information about his family situation. In all of this I would have to phrase my questions with care, for it is easy for the doctor, particularly in the active-passive relationship, to suggest to the patient an answer. For instance, if I ask the asthmatic patient, "Do you get angry just before your attack of wheezing?" he is likely to answer yes, thinking that I am suggesting anger and asthma go together. If I really wish a relatively unbiased answer, I must ask instead, "What emotion, if any, do you feel just before an asthma attack?" This still suggests to the patient that he is supposed to feel some sort of emotion, I suppose; so his answer may not be totally objective. I expect there is no real way a doctor, particularly when he appears as an authority figure to the patient, can ask a question without throwing a partial shadow of suggestion over it.

A good many patients enjoy the initial interview and are in no hurry about it, which is as it should be. Still, a doctor who is limited to some extent by a busy practice must know how to bring a rambling patient back to the matter in hand, and to bring the interview to a conclusion, all without disturbing the patient's faith and trust and feeling that the doctor has his best interests at heart.

The shaman learns early in the game, for instance, never to drum his fingers upon his desk and above all, never to glance at his watch or clock. He has lost his patient if he appears to be hurried. Nor should he interrupt the patient's responses or come in in the middle of the sentence. Even the wise "hmmmming" should be kept to a minimum. There is, as anyone can see, an art to being a shaman.

A thorough physical examination follows the initial interview, with various laboratory tests and tests for allergy. In a later interview, usually, I discuss the findings with the patient, being careful to explain their relationship to his health as clearly as I can. I want to be sure that he does not misunderstand the possibilities or, later, the importance of treatment measures. I always call the referring doctor also, for he has usually seen the patient a number of times and has a pretty good picture of his or her mental state as well as past health problems and the like. He may even be able to fill me in on family background and other relevant factors in the patient's life; such stresses, for instance, as recent death in the family, the breakup of a marriage, or, in the case of a child, the divorce of the parents.

Instructions for treatment should be as simple and as clear as possible. I provide a good many instruction sheets to my patients to minimize misunderstanding. And right about here is where I begin to meet negative responses: "What, I can't even have a bit of butter on my bread?" "You mean, not even one teensy beer?" "Oh no, Dr. Frazier! How can I get rid of Fido? He's one of the family!" The golden period of rapport between shaman and patient is apt to be diluted by lists of prescriptions and proscriptions. I can only hope to be able to arrive at a diagnosis before the patient gets his back up and to offer him a plausible explanation of his problem. If this is accomplished, his initial dismay over treatment necessities will be tempered by signs of improvement. Try as he may, it is not always possible for the allergist to bring about improvement quickly enough to suit the patient. The latter may then become depressed or angry, and either emotion may aggravate his symptoms to make matters worse. When a patient loses his trust in his shaman, it is pretty hard on the shaman, too, although I am sure that patients rarely view it from that angle. However, the shaman cannot allow his own discouragement to color his relationship with his depressed or angry patient; rather he must work to restore the patient's will to get well.

Being a shaman is often a little like being a shadow of yourself. You must step outside of your own life's experiences, in a manner of speaking, in order to remain objective toward those of your patient. Nor can you let judgment enter into your responses. Detachment yet warmth, interest, and sympathy are the orders of the day. The shaman must keep his own emotions at arm's length in order to deal with those of his troubled patient. It is not always easy, believe me.

When dealing with allergic children, the shaman also finds himself dealing with the family situation. In fact, when he has stubborn allergy symptoms to treat, he *must* deal with the family situation. In many cases, the family often need his support and help as much as the child does, for they can be anxious and perplexed, unsure of how to react to the chronically ill child, unsure of their ability to help him, and even exhausted and resentful before the demands of his illness. The first step, I think, is to be sure parents understand the nature of the child's allergy, what causes it, how it can be treated, and their role in that treatment. Then, I firmly believe that they should understand the possibility of emotional factors in their child's illness. Such factors, if they exist, usually come to light in this discussion. If the child is asthmatic, I explain the relationship of fear and anxiety to the severity of his attacks. If the child is eczematous, we discuss the damage this condition can do to his self-confidence and self-image. I can explain, without intruding into the family's privacy, that the chronically ill child needs support from parents but not smothering. I try to show the child's mother that it is possible to become so involved with the sick child as to neglect the needs of the husband or other children in the family, and that this has a rebound effect even upon the allergic child, since it breeds resentment and outright hostility. I try to explain that treating the ill child differently from his siblings not only causes family conflict, but also reinforces his illness. How do you get parents to untangle themselves from their overprotective attitudes? Mothers especially? Well, of course, you educate them well in the fundamentals of their child's illness. Often what they fear is a figment of their imaginations rather than reality. You also try to demonstrate the harm such spoiling can do the child. You hand out specific recommendations: Go out on the town once a week, but set up a plan of action with your baby-sitter in case the child becomes ill; then you can enjoy yourself without suffering undue anxiety. Take a vacation away from the child annually; begin with just a one-night stand, and gradually lengthen your holiday. Help your child develop contacts outside the family circle. Help him have a good social life on his own. This does not mean trying to buy friends and the like. It means encouraging him, helping by making the home available and pleasant for his friends, chauffeuring him when necessary, and the like. It does not mean parents arranging; it means parents encouraging.

Let's take a look at a young patient who more or less typifies the allergic youngsters I see every day. He will have asthma, for this is normally the most difficult of allergy disease for parents to deal with and, along with eczema, commonly carries the heaviest burden of emotional stress. At seven, Bobby Brown began to have mild attacks of wheezing, which usually accompanied a "cold." When these attacks increased in severity, the family doctor referred Bobby to me. He turned out to be allergic to several foods and several pollens. More than that, Bobby appeared to be suffering from concomitant emotional stresses with his peers and within the family as well.

What kind of emotional stresses can a third grader have? You have to be middle-aged and short of memory to even ask! Life is real and life is earnest, even for youngsters only eight or nine years into it. For instance, Bobby has two sisters, both younger than himself. One is only two and still needs a good deal of Mrs. Brown's attention. But Bobby is frightened by his asthma attacks, and he has become increasingly dependent upon his mother for reassurance and care. And she is just as frightened by his attacks, yet is torn between the needs of the other children and his needs. Anxious and exhausted, she is caught in a treadmill of fear for the child she loves well and the drain he is imposing on her waning energy. And she is touched by doubt . . . .

"My neighbors keep telling me that there is really nothing wrong with Bobby. That it's just nerves or that he's too highstrung. I can't really believe that. Not when I see him fight to breathe. They say he does it just to get my attention and that if I ignore him, he'll stop. It does seem that every time I need to do something for the baby, he begins to wheeze . . . ."

"And Dr. X, your family doctor, he thinks there's nothing wrong with Bobby?"

"Mercy, no! That's why we came today. Dr. X thinks he may be allergic to something about the house. But he really does start to wheeze at the most inconvenient times. Just when Bob, his father, and I plan to go out for an evening or when we have a family outing planned. He never fails. It's become a sort of family joke. And it does look, you know, Dr. Frazier, as though . . . as though, well, he does it on purpose." She states this last somewhat defiantly, as though she feels a little guilty about saying it at all.

"And this stirs up quite a bit of resentment in the family?"

"Well, yes, in a way. Bob thinks he wheezes on purpose to get his way. He even accuses me of . . . well, spoiling him, giving in to him too much. And, of course, the girls get absolutely furious with him when we had something planned and then can't do it. Why last Saturday we were halfway out the door on our way to the zoo when be began. And it was quite a bad attack. I almost had to call Dr. X."

"What happened just before the attack? Had Bobby gotten angry about something?"

She thinks a moment. "I don't think . . . no, wait, the kids were having an argument about who was going to sit up front with Bob and me, and Bob said Anna would. That it was her turn. Bobby did sulk about that, I remember. I remember I told Bob later that it would have been simpler just to let Bobby sit up front. Then we wouldn't have had all that fuss. After all, he is the oldest . . . ."

"Hmmmm. How is he doing at school?"

"That's another worrisome problem. He's not doing too well. He's already been absent almost a month this year and he's gotten behind."

"And his relations with his peers? The other boys?"

She frowns and looks thoughtful. "Not good, I'm afraid. They seem to have nicknamed him 'The Whistler' and 'Steamboat Bill.' I hear them calling such things to him as they go by when he's playing out in the yard. And he hasn't any friends really. He can't really join in their games. He begins to wheeze almost at once when he exerts. I do have to keep him rather close . . . ." Her voice trails off and she stares at her hands folded in her lap.

"Hmmmm." (Shamans are much given to "hmmmming," but as I said, we must keep it to a minimum lest patients take it as a sign of perplexity.)

"He gets picked on a lot," she continues in a troubled voice. "Even the gym teacher at school is always after him for slouching and because I have to keep sending notes to have him excused from PE classes after his attacks. Most of what they do anyway is too strenuous for him. I've had to pick him up at the nurse's office a number of times after gym class."

She sighs. "I guess I have to admit, Doctor, that I'm getting a bit worn down by all this, especially because neither he nor I get many good nights sleep any more. I find myself being, well, short with him sometimes. Sometimes even when he is wheezing, and then I feel guilty and so I give in to him. And I give in to him too much, I know, because his attacks frighten me so. He . . . he actually can't get his breath and I'm so afraid that he will . . . will suffocate. Oh, I know I shouldn't let him have his way so often. I give in to him on things I'd never consider letting the girls get away with. And that upsets them, of course. Oh. It's a mess. And I really don't know what to do. I really don't, Doctor!"

There is real desperation in her voice now. It is time to stop sage hmmming, time to apply instead some reassuring, humanistic remedies. Let us tackle this problem.

First we must recognize and deal with Bobby's anxiety about his asthma attacks. They frighten him, as they frighten his mother. The older he grows, the greater his awareness of anxiety and of death. It is strange, but often infants suffering asthma attacks may lie on their backs, wheezing badly, but playing with a toy all the while and smiling happily. It may be that they have a different breathing pattern from the older child's and are thus not so much bothered; but it may also be that the absence of anxiety has something to do with it. Anxiety, as we have seen in earlier chapters, plays the heavy in asthma. For example, I once hypnotized a patient with asthma whose attack was serious enough to call for hospitalization. I thought my hypnotic powers had done the trick when she became relaxed and comfortable, but when I listened to her chest, I found that she was wheezing just as badly as before. Now, however, she didn't seem upset by it. Outwardly, her asthma was greatly relieved. Inwardly, it was far from it.

In any case, as Bobby became more anxious and frightened by his asthma, his dependence on his mother increased. And because she, too, was frightened by his attacks, she encouraged that dependence.

It is altogether natural for a frightened child to turn to his mother so, and altogether natural that she should do all she can to reassure and help him. Therefore, the fears of both mother and child must be alleviated. But how?

We treat Bobby's asthma and try to bring it under control. We use medications and avoidance measures to accomplish this, and, if possible, we try to desensitize him to the allergens causing his problem. We make sure that parents and youngster both have a working knowledge of his problem and of the role anxiety is playing in aggravating his symptoms. We teach Bobby breathing exercises (see Appendix K, page 245) and relaxation exercises (see Appendix I, page 240) as a means of helping alleviate the severity and frequency of his attacks. We reassure the parents and the boy as to the eventual outcome of his asthma, and we suggest with all the power of our shamanship that he will soon be well.

Then we turn our attention to other matters within the family and in Bobby's experiences at school and among his peers, all of which may be very important to that hoped-for "cure."

For instance, Bobby may have developed considerable additional anxiety about his mother's somewhat ambivalent feelings toward him, her overprotection vacillating with feelings of resentment and/or rejection. He was literally a monkey wrench thrown into the family machinery, and he has sensed it. It is easy to imagine his sisters on the day of the aborted trip to the zoo, "Oh, he spoils everything!" and his mother calling off the baby-sitter in some exasperation as his father fumes, "You'd think for just once we could get out of this house!" Youngsters have an uncanny way of sensing even what may not be fully or candidly expressed.

Bobby's problems do not stop with anxiety. Because his play and sports activity have been limited by his asthma, he has found himself singled out even at his early age as a "sissy," the ineffectual male so despised in our somewhat aggressive society. And that hurts! Bobby has soon discovered how much it hurts in an endless assortment of situations, including gym classes where he sits on the sidelines, his "excuse" clutched in his hand. There is adult authority in the shape of a gruff and unsympathetic gym teacher who announces for all the class to hear, "If you'd get out there and play a little football, Brown, it might make a man out of you!" By the time he had experienced much of this, Bobby's self-confidence and self-esteem would doubtlessly be lower than the proverbial snake's belly.

And what goes on in the classroom may be just as hurtful as what goes on in the gym or out on the playing field. Frequent absences from school keep Bobby struggling to catch up. Make-up tests dominate his after-school hours. Surely more than one teacher has indicated exasperation, too, with the endless parade of "excuses" from home: "Please be sure Bobby does not sit near a window. Drafts bring on his asthma." "Please excuse Robert half an hour early. He has an appointment with the doctor." "Please give Bobby this pill twice a day." If the teacher does not understand the necessity behind these constant instructions, she is apt to find them vexing.

It would be a wonder if young Bobby Brown, burdened by chronic illness that frightens him badly, by pressures at school and among his peers, and by family conflict with himself at its center, were not considerably stressed emotionally. However, he has discovered a sure way of his own to get back a bit. He has found that he can bring the world to his feet whenever he begins to gasp and wheeze. His family will rally around him, concern on their faces. Teachers will turn pale and send him immediately to the school nurse. Even the gym teacher will grow nervous. He can even command instant attention and respect of a sort from his peers. His sisters are awed. His mother can't do enough to comfort him. His father brings home presents to make up for his suffering. He is, for the duration of his symptoms and shortly thereafter, the center of attention and the object of lavish care and affection. Small wonder that even though his own struggles to breathe frighten and exhaust him, he finds his asthma rewarding. It is something of a paradox that this chronic illness that is causing him so many problems and so much grief should also provide him a place in the sun!

This brief scenario presents what is probably a common adaption to chronic allergy. What do we do about it?

We have pretty much covered this field in earlier pages, so will only touch on it briefly now. First, Bobby must "unlearn" using his allergy as a crutch. He needs reinforcement in a different direction.

"Accentuate the positive," I tell Bobby's parents. "Refrain from rewarding his suffering because, you see, it indicates to him that it pays to be ill. If he can win, say, a new bike by simply having an asthma attack, he will learn that asthma has a payoff. What you need to do instead is to reinforce the importance of staying healthy, of managing his own problem. Reward, for instance, given periods of being asthma-free. Reward his taking on of responsibility in avoiding allergens and chilling and the like."

I hasten to elaborate on this theme, lest they conclude that Bobby has been hustling them all this time.

"Please understand that I'm not saying that Bobby consciously choses to have an asthma attack to get his own way. When he is frustrated, he may become emotionally upset, and this may precipitate an attack. But then so may getting chilled. Even so, he has to be disciplined as a normal child is to remain a normal child. He cannot be allowed to rule the family, for that isn't fair to the rest of you and it isn't fair to him. Perhaps common sense here is the answer and a bit of preventive action. When you feel that he is becoming emotionally upset, give him his asthma medication. But above all, don't teach him to use asthma by rewarding it."

"There is a recent theory," I continue "that suggests that the allergic individual's cells become conditioned to respond to stressful stimuli as well as to actual allergens in much the same way Pavlov's dogs learned to salivate to the sound of a bell as they did naturally to the sight or smell of food. In much the same way, this theory proposes, after so many reactions to an allergen in conjunction with emotional stress, the emotional stress alone may trigger the allergic reaction in some people. Not all allergic persons, but those, I suppose, who are somewhat susceptible to suggestion. I would think that this might be very true when the allergic reaction has been rewarded. Thus, if you feel lonely and depressed and can immediately gain love and attention in abundance by having an attack of asthma, well . . . it is easy to understand how asthma can become a habitual response to emotional discomfort. Even the common cold appears to turn up not only in response to a bug but also in response to emotional turmoil. Our minds are adept at finding ways out of emotional distress. Escape hatches, so to speak.

"To be more specific, do not be afraid to discipline Bobby as you do his sisters. Try not to reward his asthma, but love him well. Don't make him feel set apart or different. In fact, he should be encouraged to participate in normal games and sport. He should learn that if he begins to wheeze he should stop immediately and rest. If you find that he cannot play football, and he may well be able to once medication, diet, and avoidance measures stabilize his allergy, you know, then encourage him to take up a less strenuous sport. Encourage him to learn and to excel in some athletic endeavor so that he can gain the respect he needs: self-respect and the respect of his peers.

"By the same token, if asthma forces him to miss too many school days, it's very important that he not fall behind. His self-esteem and self-confidence are equally important in this area also. Arrange for a temporary tutor or make some accomodation with the school. Anxiety about lagging behind can only aggravate his asthma. He needs encouragement in his schoolwork and recognition, not an educational put-down. You'd be surprised how severe asthma can get when a patient gives up on himself. And this can happen even to a child.

"There are a few things Bobby will need to do that may be a bit special other than his avoidance measures. He should get plenty of rest and not become unduly fatigued. He should also dress warmly in cold weather and avoid catching cold, if that's possible."

I believe that the Browns leave my office resolved to view the future differently. I hope that I have relieved them of some of their anxieties and given them a working blueprint for Bobby and his asthma.

There are many variations on the Bobby Brown theme and many varieties of emotional problems that may be encountered among asthmatic children. Sometimes I am confronted by a severely asthmatic child so hostile, so anxious, so rejected that he cowers like a cornered animal in my office. Often, even though the parents put on quite an act about caring for the child, the evidences of neglect are there: bad teeth; dirty, broken fingernails; untidy clothes. Nor are these children from poor families. Frequently, in such cases, the child's emotional stress within the family is so great that I recommend "parentectomy," the separation of the child from the family situation for a year or two. There are special institutions, homes is a better word, where such children are treated not only for the physical aspects of their asthma, but for their emotional problems as well. Often enough, removal from the family and its conflicts is enough to relieve both asthma and emotional tension. One such "home away from home," Children's Asthma Research Institute and Hospital, in Denver, reports that some 80 percent of the children entering with intractable asthma and who have stayed for periods of 18 to 24 months leave requiring greatly decreased amounts of medication to lead a normal life. They report that some of the boys are even able to play football and that once-bedridden asthmatic children can again participate in competitive sports.

A miracle? Well, perhaps. In a way.

Since by adulthood we tend to become pretty set in our ways, it is a bit more difficult for the shaman to lay it on his grown-up allergic patients. Yet, I never cease to be astonished at how therapeutic just "talking it out" seems to be. Emotional problems brought into the light of day can be comprehended and approached. And insight into the problem is the first great step toward solving it. A large dose of reassurance can go a long way in relieving the anxiety that is aggravating allergy symptoms. Adult asthmatic patients are as frightened and anxious about their struggles for breath as children, and eczematous patients fear that they will spend a lifetime being disfigured. Combine the catharsis of talking it out with reassurance, a clear understanding of the mechanism of the allergy, a measure of common sense, and a pleasant prognosis, and often enough the load of emotional stress is lightened. As that load is diminished, nine times out of ten, so are allergic symptoms.

This is not to say that the shaman need not be wily on occasion. Some allergic adults can be pretty tricky, difficult, bullheaded, stubborn, and some do not wish to give up their allergy. Fortunately, this last category is very rare. But when I am confronted by so crippled a patient, I know I must refer him to a different kind of shaman, a psychiatrist. The bullheaded patient is a horse of a different color. Unfortunately, the older we grow, the more committed we become to this and that, particularly our little pleasures, our pleasing vices. Smoking is a case in point.

"Doc, you gotta give me something so's I can breathe better. I can (gasp) hardly smoke a cigarette anymore."

Do I exaggerate?

I wish I did. Alas, many an asthmatic patient is so hooked on cigarettes that he won't give them up even if they kill him. Which they might. But as we know from the Surgeon General's less-than-successful efforts, it seldom does much good to warn or even to try to frighten the confirmed smoker. Some medical men think smoking—other than mild, social, going-along-with-the-crowd type—indicates emotional deprivation, that it is used as a shield against frustration, perhaps even guilt. Whatever it represents emotionally, smoking, like other addictions (alcohol, heavy drugs, and the like) is not given up easily, no doubt because it does satisfy some powerful psychological need. An allergist's approach to an allergic patient, particularly the asthmatic patient, must take this possibility into account, for the patient, if he is to be well, must break out of the habit any way he can. (See Appendix G, page 237 for some suggestions on how to quit smoking.)

As we have noted, asthma and eczema have been linked with difficulty in weeping, even in the face of profound grief. They have been likened to a "suppressed cry." I have an asthmatic and eczematous patients whose symptoms have diminished markedly when they could open the floodgates of their sorrows. These are often the people who, too controlled, seem to benefit most by talking it out, from sympathy and understanding, from the doctor's just being there to listen. Grief often enters our lives with shocking suddenness. Sometimes we are too stunned even to weep. The old custom of openly wailing at funerals, of tearing of clothes and the like, may have been unsightly, but it seems to have been an excellent way of expressing one of our most powerful of human emotions. In our busy society we are, I think, too mannerly, too hipped on being cool, too removed from the elemental need to weep or to laugh, to shout or to sing, to dance or to lie dreaming in the sun. We tend to bottle up our profound emotions to maintain our "image." Strong silent types that we are, we seem to prefer to suffer the consequences of illness, for illness will be the result when we keep the cork in the bottle for any length of time. It is strange that custom should so often dictate harshly against the needs of the psyche.

One of the most difficult of all adult allergic patients to treat is the depressed individual, the person who arrives at the shaman's office saying, "You can't help me, Doctor. I've been to others. I've tried all sorts of things, but nothing helps." A patient who has given up on himself is a hard nut to crack, and sometimes when depression is deep, it is also dangerous. When I believe this to be the case, again I do not hesitate to refer such a patient to a psychiatrist, for literally the patient's life may be at stake. Whether the depression is a result of chronic and limiting asthma or eczema or other allergy, or of some preceding life experiences, makes little difference in the prognosis of his symptoms, for his prognosis will be poor as long as he firmly believes that he cannot be helped. Fortunately, again, such patients are very rare.

How does the shaman overcome the apathy, the loneliness, the withdrawal from life of the less-than-dangerously-depressed patient? It isn't easy. A somewhat classic example is the woman at menopause. Usually her children are grown and often as not gone from the home. Thus, she feels that her life's work, her usefulness is over. She also feels that her attractiveness as a woman is diminished. She has neither enough to do nor enough to occupy her mind. Lonely, bored, at loose ends, she may take refuge in illness and depression. What can the shaman do? He can listen to her tale of woe first. Then he can do his best to make her comprehend the change that has occurred not only in her body, but in her life situation. Then he can accentuate the positive. "Look," he can say, "you are free at last to pursue whatever you wish. You have done a great job, accomplished a great thing. You have raised your fine family and launched them into the world. That is an accomplishment of the first magnitude. Nothing could be more important. You have done all this at the expense of your own needs, your own ambitions. So, now it is time to live for yourself. Go back to those things that once interested you. Pick up your dreams again. Take up a career, a sport, a hobby. Feel no guilt for time spent now on yourself, for you have done your job and for 20 or 30 years you have selflessly worked for others. Now, go out and live for yourself."

This is grand advice. But when a woman has spent all these years in one job, it's not quite so simple to lay it all down and begin anew. Yet, to be happy this is what many women must consider doing in their middle years. And they will need encouragement, support, and reassurance, not only from the shaman, but from their husbands as well. The shaman would do well to be sure husbands understand this need. Thus, the shaman not only treats the allergy of such patients, but must needs do his best to treat their emotional turmoil in finding themselves abruptly "abandoned."

In general, the emotional stresses of the allergic patients I treat are of the garden variety—marital difficulties, personal problems of grief and anxiety, hostility and guilt, loneliness and depression. Often enough, such stress is greatly diminished when their allergic symptoms are alleviated by standard medical treatment and by a little shamanship on my part. I encourage talking out as best I can; I listen sympathetically; I try to help them gain insight into the problem; I encourage; I support; I offer limited and wary advice, for the solution must lie with them. Those who are obviously very tense, I try to relax, either with mild tranquilizers or by my own approach. I try to give faith in a cure. When I say, "You're okay" or "You'll live to be a hundred," I want them to believe it.

So, to sum up all this: is there an allergy personality–a certain type of person likely to develop allergy, his character so clearly delineated that we can predict that the chances are good that he will? I don't really think there is. I believe that the role of emotional stress is very great in allergy. I believe it can trigger and aggravate allergy symptoms. I also believe that allergy itself, especially if improperly managed, can play a very large role in creating emotional stress and in developing many maladaptive personality facets. To know which comes first, emotional stress or allergy illness, may be of vital importance in allergy research, but in treating the individual patient it doesn't much matter. You can be a good shaman, a very decent witch doctor, even if you are a little unscientific about it.

APPENDIX A
How to Keep an Allergen-free House and Bedroom

Preparation and Maintenance of a Dust-free House

House dust is the fine dust which is formed by the aging of materials which make up household articles, furniture, and clothing. It is the fine lint and dust from mattresses, pillows, upholstered furniture, drapes, curtains, rugs, bedspreads, blankets, quilts, comforters, closets, chests, drawers, books, papers, sweaters, and other clothing. Furniture and furnishings are likely to have much lint. Dust develops in stored articles and in furniture as they become older. During the aging process the substance composing these articles deteriorates into a fine dust.

Street dust is entirely different from house dust. Your cooperation in controlling the amount of house dust which you inhale will be of tremendous benefit to you. We cannot urge you too strongly the importance of carrying out the house-dust avoidance instructions which follow.

Bedroom

1. The room must be completely emptied, just as if you were moving. Give the room a thorough cleaning and scrubbing to eliminate all traces of dust. Clean walls; wash them down if possible. Scrub the woodwork, floors, baseboards, closets, etc. Every inch of exposed or hidden surface must be spic and span. Floors or linoleum should then be oiled or waxed. Linoleum if used, should be cemented to the floor. Rag rugs may be used on the floor. These should be washed weekly.
2. Cleaning should be done only when the patient is out of the room.
3. Outside the room, clean every inch of the bed. Scrub the bed and open-coil springs. Bed and coil springs should be cleaned every two weeks. If the same mattress and box springs are to be used, each should be encased with an allergic dust-proof cover. Merely clean with a damp, soapy cloth

and wipe dry. If you have a sleep sentry dust-proof mattress and box springs no special covers are required. Ordinary pillows must be made dust proof with special coverings, which may be obtained from Allergen Proof Encasings, Inc., 4060 Superior Ave., Cleveland 3, Ohio or 3 Park Place, New York 7, N.Y., with zippers sealed with adhesive tape for maximum protection. A dust-free pillow may be used in the room with special coverings. Rubber foam pillows may be used. If two beds are to be used in the room, both must be prepared identically.

4. Use only freshly laundered linens, washable cotton spreads, woolen blankets (not the fuzzy kind). If you are sensitive to wool, use ordinary cotton blankets. Blankets and spreads should be washed at least once a month. Do not use comforters and avoid blankets that have not been washed. Plain light curtains or venetian blinds may be used on the windows. Wash them weekly. Scrubbed wooden or metal chairs, or chairs covered with leather or leatherette, may be used in this room. Upholstered furniture is taboo.

5. Clothing must be stored outside the room. Dressing and undressing should be done in another room.
   Keep all pets out of the room and the house, especially dogs and cats. Canaries, parrots, and pigeons are not allowed as pets.
   Screens, ventilators, or anything that helps keep out dust and pollens is desirable. Use only insecticides and cosmetics approved by your doctor.

6. The temperature of this room, when occupied, should always be above 65 degrees, particularly at night. Determine the temperature of this room by means of a wall thermometer.
   Steam or hot water heat is preferable to hot air heat. An electric heater or a good gas heater may be used. If furnace heat outlets exist, a dust filter must be installed and the filter changed frequently. When not in use, furnace pipe outlets should be sealed with a dust-proof fabric held intact with adhesive. Holes or cracks in the floor or walls should be sealed.

7. This room should be cleaned daily and thoroughly cleaned weekly. Do it while the patient is out of the room. If the patient must clean her own room, a gauze mask should be worn. After cleaning, shut the windows and doors for an hour or two before the patient is ready to occupy the room. Keep the doors and windows of the room closed as much as possible. Do not permit drafts and cross ventilation in this room.

Other Parts of the House

8. For housecleaning, oil mops and vacuum cleaners should be used. Do not use brooms and dusters. Keep patient out of the house while it is being

cleaned. The house should be well aired before the patient returns to it after it is cleaned.

9. Upholstered furniture throughout the house and rugs should be vacuumed frequently; daily, if possible. Whenever possible do not permit the patient to sit or lie on upholstered furniture.
10. Do not permit the use of stuffed toys. Toys should be wooden, rubber, plastic, or iron. If impractical to keep patient out of the house while it is being cleaned, have her wear a mask at that time. A practical and inexpensive mask and refills is the Martindale Protective Mask, made by the Martindale Electronic Co., Box 617, Edgewater Branch, Cleveland, Ohio.
11. Dust catchers should be removed from the house.
12. Contact with irritating odors, such as leaking stoves, refrigerators, kerosene lamps, heaters, fresh paint, camphor, tar, smoke from smudge fires or burning trash, should be avoided.
13. Be sure that all clothes and bedclothes that have been stored are well aired or cleaned before using them.
14. Patient should not handle objects that are dusty, such as books, boxes, or clothing that has been stored in cases, closets or storerooms, trunks, chests, or attics over a long period of time. Patient should not go into attics, closets, or storerooms, or rummage in drawers.
15. Do not permit patient to wear linty materials, such as sweaters, particularly angora sweaters and knitted goods. If sweaters must be used, be sure that they have been washed or cleaned several times and most of the lint is removed.
16. Patient should not use knitting or embroidery wool.
17. Patient should never be in rooms whose temperature is below 65 degrees. Patient should never dust the erasers in school.

While the above directions may seem difficult at first, experience plus habit will make them simple, and the results will be well worth the effort.

APPENDIX B
How to Combat Mold and Mildew

Places Where Molds Are Found

1. Gardens
2. Farms
3. In occupations of: (A) carpenters, (B) bakers, (C) florists, (D) farmers, (E) paper hangers, (F) mill workers, and (G) workers in mattress upholstery
4. Summer cottages
5. Grain bins
6. Potted plants and leaves
7. Some foods: (A) cheese, (B) bread, (C) yeast, and (D) decayed foods
8. Damp closets
9. Mattresses
10. Some grasses and weeds
11. Shoes and clothing in closets.

Molds grow best in warm, moist places and grow on nearly anything except metals. They grow on feathers, trees, plants, and cellulose, and they may be outside or inside the house. They occur all year round but some molds have a seasonal incidence. Some molds are found more just after frost occurs and when the leaves fall.

To Avoid Molds

1. Avoid damp basements.
2. Avoid being out in a storm.

3. Avoid occupations where molds are found such as: paper hanging, mill working, mattress upholstering, antique and furniture dealing, etc.
4. Avoid foods with molds on them such as cheese, moldy bread, yeast, and decayed foods.
5. Follow dust and feather control measures.
6. Keep luggage dry and waxed.
7. Change furnace filters.
8. Check drainage systems.
9. Avoid cleaning out leaves in the fall and cutting grass in the summer.
10. If you use a summer cottage, have it aired out well before going inside.

APPENDIX C
How to Avoid Bees, Yellowjackets, Wasps, and Hornets if Allergic

1. *Known habits.*

These insects are outdoors from April to November. Wasps, especially, often crawl into houses as cold weather approaches. Wet weather often angers bees and makes them inclined to sting because rain washes pollen from flowers.

Bees make their homes in hollow tree trunks, posts (bumblebees in crevices above and below ground). They feed on clover and flowers.

Yellowjackets make their homes in holes in the ground, posts, stumps, rock walls. They feed on rotten fruit and love watermelon juice, melting ice cream, fruit punch. They are frequently found around the bases of fruit trees, picnic areas, garbage cans.

Wasps make their nests under eaves and windowsills. They feed on the same kind of goodies favored by their cousins, the yellowjackets, and are found in similar places.

Hornets make their homes in papier-mâché football-sized (often) nests hung from tree limbs, in bushes, or in long grass.

2. *Avoid attracting.*

Do *not* use scented lotions, perfumes, shampoos, and the like during the insect season.

Do *not* wear bright colors and flowery prints, floppy clothing, bright metal costume jewelry or belt buckles, suede or leather (animal odors seem to attract and annoy), or sandals (too much exposed foot).

Do wear shoes, a headscarf if hair is long (bees, etc., can become entangled in long hair and may sting), and smooth-finished fabrics of light color (tan, green, white, khaki).

Do shake out any clothing left undisturbed for any length of time before putting it on. Many a man has harbored a wasp or its ilk in a pants' leg or sleeve.

3. *Remove nests in immediate environment.*

Begin this chore with first warm weather and patrol and destroy until after first

fall frosts. Nests are easier to tackle when in construction stage or still small. However, no allergic person should attempt this chore himself. Call an exterminator or let a nonallergic person handle it.
To get rid of bees, call nearest beekeeper.
To get rid of yellowjacket nests pour gas, kerosene down holes *at night.* Do not light, for the fumes do the trick.
To get rid of wasps knock nests down with a broom handle (and run).
To get rid of hornets call the fire department.

4. *Wear a medical warning tag such as Medic Alert at all times.*
Contact Medic Alert Foundation, Turlock, California 95380, or National Identification Company, 3955 Oneida Street, Denver, Colorado 80207.

APPENDIX D
How to Manage an Elimination Diet

At the end of each initial work-up, the patient is given a list of foods to avoid as much as possible and one to avoid completely. In about 10–14 days the patient is asked to start adding these foods back to the diet, one at a time, along with the foods she is already eating. The patient should start with the food that she feels most necessary to resume a well-balanced diet. After choosing the food she will start with, she is asked to eat a small amount of this food the first day, and to increase the amounts gradually until she has eaten this particular food for five days, if this is a food that the patient finds difficult to eat for five days in fairly large amounts. In the case of a child, three days of trying a food is usually sufficient, as it is difficult to make a child eat some foods five days in a row. After the trial period for this food is completed, they are asked to omit this food for two days to allow it to get out of their system. Then they may have this particular food any time they want it, as it is apparently not a troublemaker. Then they should go on to another food, trying it the same way.

The patient should watch for a flare-up of allergy symptoms while trying a new food. Food allergy can affect a person in many ways, by sneezing, an increase in nasal congestion or postnasal drainage, headaches, vomiting, diarrhea, or skin rash. If you have a flare-up of symptoms, before you blame the food, think of other things that might have brought on the symptoms, such as a visit to a home where there are dogs or cats, or being around a large number of potted plants, or a change in weather, or a visit to a dusty home, or being around where old books or newspapers have been stored and are collecting dust and molds. If there is no explanation for the symptoms, the patient is asked to stop eating the food that she had been trying, and wait for two days before starting on a new food. In a month, the patient should go back and retry the food that she thought caused the flare-up of symptoms. If the same flare-up occurs the second time of trying this food, then the patient should avoid this food for a year before retrying it.

Our patients are asked to follow through with this elimination diet, as food testing is not reliable, and the only way to tell if one has food allergies is through trying the foods and seeing which ones cause trouble.

ELIMINATION DIET
and
GENERAL RULES FOR FEEDING AN ALLERGIC PATIENT

DR. CLAUDE A. FRAZIER **ASHEVILLE, N. C.** **DOCTOR'S PARK**

1. **When a food is added to the patient's diet, the food must be eaten daily for 5 days. Eat a small portion the first day, and a large portion at least twice a day for the next 4 days.**
2. **Introduce one food at a time into the diet of the patient, and do not add any other food for 7 days. The purpose is to see how each particular food affects the allergy, and of course if it makes it worse, it should be omitted. No new food may be considered as a part of the patient's regular diet until the trial period of 5 days has been observed. If the food causes no symptoms within 5 days of trial, it may be added to the permitted diet after eliminating 2 more days.**
3. **Add one of the foods listed to the patient's present diet every 7 days.**
4. **Any food which causes any symptoms should be stopped promptly. Wait until the symptoms caused by the food on trial have subsided completely before trying the next food (2 days).**
5. **It is not necessary to try any food you do not like, or do not want to add to the normal diet.**
6. **All foods should be thoroughly cooked before being fed to the patient.**
7. **Unless you are certain of the ingredients in a certain dish, do not give it to the patient.**
8. **During the first year of life, only a few foods should be given.**
9. **When a new food is offered, it should be a single food, and not mixtures. Some prepared vegetables have more than one vegetable present, and if the allergy became worse with the mixed foods, we would not know the single offending food.**
10. **Excessively large amounts of any food should be avoided. This also applies to milk.**
11. **No patient should be starved because of his allergy, and allowed to get into a state of malnutrition.**
12. **Keep a record of the effect of each food added in the chart below.**

DATE	FOOD ADDED	EFFECT

APPENDIX E

How to Avoid Aspirin-related Foods and Additives

Since aspirin allergy can be severe, many allergists recommend that such patients avoid not only the drug itself but the following foods that contain an ingredient of aspirin-salicylate:

almonds	blackberries
apples	boysenberries
apple cider	currants
apricots	gooseberries
raspberries	peaches
strawberries	plums
prunes	oranges
grapes	raisins
cucumbers	pickles
tomatoes	cloves
oil of wintergreen	

The last item, oil of wintergreen, turns up in unexpected places, such as toothpastes, mouthwashes, and the like. A yellow dye, Tartrazine, is so closely related to aspirin chemically that it also seems to be able to cause a reaction in aspirin-sensitive individuals. This dye is used to color all kinds of foods from soft drinks to baked goods.

APPENDIX F
How Not to Scratch

Roerig Pfizer, a division of Pfizer Pharmaceuticals of New York, put out an attractive and helpful booklet entitled *All About Itching.* With their kind permission I would like to reproduce here the section "Things You Can Do to Help Reduce Itching":

There are several steps that you can take to help minimize the discomfort of the itching associated with your skin condition. However, not all of these steps may be applicable to your particular situation. Following is a list of things that you can do to help reduce itching; note and follow those that your physician has checked off.

_ Scratch as little as possible and not too vigorously.
Remember, vigorous scratching can lead to a worsening of your skin condition and possibly infection, as well as actually cause an intensification of the pruritus (itching).

_ Avoid irritating agents.
Avoid contact with irritating agents, including strong alkaline or perfumed soaps, chemicals, dyes, etc.; cotton clothing is preferable to that made of wool or nylon.

_ Avoid aggravating situations.
Stress and anxiety may cause renewed outbreaks of your symptoms and may lead to uncontrolled scratching.

_ Keep cool.
Avoid getting overheated as well as sudden changes in temperature; excessive perspiration is a known trigger in pruritis. Cold compresses, baths or showers may help control itching.

_ Try applications of heat via very hot water.
Paradoxically, some cases of localized pruritis respond to applications of very hot water (120 to 130°F); apply with wash cloth or place affected area under running water for brief periods; DO NOT ATTEMPT A BATH OR SHOWER AT THESE TEMPERATURES.

_ Avoid drying out your skin.
Excessive bathing and use of strong soaps tend to remove important natural oils on your skin and thus aggravates pruritus.
Avoid exposure to cold and wind.
Avoid exposure to low humidity environments.

_ Keep physically and mentally active.
Bouts of pruritus occur most often when we have little else to occupy our mind and least frequently when our attentions are diverted elsewhere; however, avoid overheating and fatigue, both of which tend to increase itching.

_ For patients with an allergic skin condition; keep a diary.
Carry a small diary or other means of notetaking with you and record what happened *immediately preceding* any worsening of your condition as a way of pinpointing causative factors.

_ Follow instructions regarding topical medications faithfully.
Do not alter or stop your course of therapy without consulting (your doctor) first.

_ Follow instructions regarding internal medications faithfully.
Do not alter or stop your course of therapy without consulting (your doctor) first.

APPENDIX G
How Not to Smoke

1. Begin by asking yourself why you smoke. Write down your reasons and consider them well. Then consider the risk you are taking as a smoker. A pack-a-day man has 20 times the chance of dying of lung cancer as the nonsmoker and loses, on the average, six-and-one-half years of his lifetime. And so on with all the well-publicized facts and figures. The smoker knows them well. He just doesn't pay any attention. Pay attention now and weigh such statistics carefully, for it is now your own life you are considering; it is your own choice of how and when you will die that you are making.

2. So, now that you have chosen to give up cigarettes, make up your mind that you *do* possess the willpower necessary to do it.

3. If you are a heavy smoker, it is wiser to give up cigarettes cold turkey. Now, a light smoker can probably get away with cutting down and phasing out, but a heavy smoker has little chance that way. He does best to gird up his willpower, pick a day, and stop.

4. Repeat constantly in your mind, under your breath, or shout, "I will not smoke!" or "I do not wish to smoke!" Keep it up for the first smokeless ten days. Remind yourself over and over again that *you* are the master here; your intelligence *is* in control. When the craving becomes powerful, look at a clock or your watch. You can keep from reaching for that cigarette for one moment. Better than that, you will be surprised to find that after the third moment comes and goes, your craving has diminished. It is a question of hanging in there for just those few revolutions of a sweep second hand or those all but imperceptible jerks of the minute hand.

5. Drink lots of water from quitting day forward. Water, fruit juice, milk—liquid helps pass the nicotine out of your body. One doctor recommends that you drink one or two glasses upon first rising, two glasses of water between breakfast and lunch, and two more during the afternoon.

Do not drink coffee, tea, or other stimulant drinks. Especially do *not* drink alcoholic beverages, including wine and beer. Alcohol, as is well known, diminishes willpower. You don't need that at a time like this!

6. Get plenty of rest. Put off partying for the first five to ten days after you kick the habit, for fatigue is the enemy of good nerves and a strong will.

7. Mealtime can be double trouble. Do *not* overeat. Do *not* eat spicy foods, rich foods, fried foods, sweet foods. All these can affect the nervous system and increase irritation and general feelings of unhappiness. *Do* eat fresh fruit, vegetables, fish, whole grain breads and cereals. The vitamin B complex is essential to healthy nerves. Consult your doctor about taking vitamin B supplement or help yourself daily to one or two tablespoons of wheat germ or take one or two tablespoons of brewer's yeast.

8. Often that last forkful at mealtime brings you to the moment of truth. You are happily, pleasurably full and your hand begins to reach for that after-dinner cigarette. Jump up quickly. Now do something. Either chew gum (sugarless) or nibble on an apple or take a mint. Don't sit down and relax. Go to your workshop, do something that occupies the mind, or, best of all, take a walk and increase your intake of oxygen, which in turn increases the power of your brain and that all-important willpower.

9. Specific things that will help:
   - a mild tranquilizer prescribed by your doctor
   - sugarless chewing gum
   - cloves
   - Chinese ginger
   - mints
   - fruits (fresh and raisins)
   - vigorous exercise
   - fresh air and deep breathing
   - games, crossword puzzles, jigsaws, movies
   - anniversary gifts to yourself after the first ten days without a cigarette, the first month, the second, and so on until you forget that you ever were a smoker

10. Keep your guard up! The cigarette habit lies just below the surface of your control and can explode back into being instantly. It takes a long time to *extinguish* a habit once it is firmly formed. Give it time and take nothing for granted. You will have to work at it, but it will be worth every effort you make.

APPENDIX H
How to Avoid Pollens

Tree, grass, and weed pollens have their season in most of the United States, and only in the far south are in the air on a year-round basis. Knowledge of these general seasons can help in planning avoidance measures.

Tree pollens are usually in the air from March through mid-June.

Elm	February-April, and usually begins tree pollen season April 1-15 on the eastern seaboard
Birch	April-May April 15-May 15 on eastern seaboard
Oak	April-May May 15-June 1 on eastern seaboard
Hickory	May-June and usually ends tree pollen season June 1-15 on eastern seaboard

Grass pollens are in season generally from May through July.

Timothy	July-August
Orchard	June-July
Bermuda	May-September
Red top	June-September

Weeds are generally pollinating from August into the fall, with ragweed leading the pack from mid-August through September.

There are only two states that can be considered pollen-free, Alaska and Hawaii.

APPENDIX I
How to Relax*

Relaxation Training Script
Modified Jacobsonian Method

Make yourself comfortable, legs extended, hands resting in your lap or at your sides. Be sure you are as comfortable as possible. Now close your eyes. Make a tight fist with both hands. Squeeze very tightly so that your muscles tremble somewhat. Hold it very tightly. Very tightly. (5 seconds.) Now relax, relax your hands completely, all at once. Just let them go limp. Notice the difference between the muscles when they are tense and how they feel as relaxation flows through them (10″). All right, now tense the same muscles again. Squeeze hard, very hard (5″) and relax. Very limp. Notice again the difference between tense muscles and relaxed muscles, and how they feel becoming more and more relaxed. You may feel a sense of warmth within your muscles as they get really relaxed (10″). All right, once more, squeeze, squeeze hard (5″) and relax, relax completely–no tension, completely relaxed (10″). Good, now do the upper part of your arms leaving your hands in place. When I tell you to, tense the muscles in the top part of both arms. You may feel some tension in your shoulders and maybe in the bottom part of your arms at the same time, but concentrate on your upper arms–pay attention to the tenseness in your upper arms–OK, tense your upper arm muscles, tightly, very tightly (5″), now relax, relax your arms completely. Notice the similarity in the feeling as relaxation flows through your arms–no tension, (10″)–it is important that you pay attention to this feeling so that you learn what tense muscles feel like–so that you can later relax these muscles again by noting when you have gotten rid of the tension, that same feeling of no muscle tension. OK, do the upper arm muscles again. Hands still in place, tense your upper arm muscles tightly, very tightly (5″) and relax, relax completely; very limp, warm and relaxed (10″).

*Courtesy of CARIH, The Children's Asthma Research Institute and Hospital, 1999 Julian Street, Denver, Colorado 80204.

Good, now relax the muscles in the upper part of your face. Tense these muscles by frowning very hard, closing your eyes tightly and wrinkling your nose. Go ahead, tense them very tightly, feel the tension, very tightly, (5″) and relax, let go completely. Again feel the relaxation flow through the upper part of your face (10″). Do them once more. Tense up, frown hard, close your eyes tightly, wrinkle your nose, very tightly (5″) and relax–relax completely, no tension, warm and relaxed, completely relaxed (10″). Good, the next muscles to do are in your cheeks and jaw. You can tense these muscles by pulling the corners of your mouth back as far as possible and clinching your teeth, go ahead, pull tightly, feel the tension, (5″) and relax–relax completely. Again notice the relaxation flowing through the muscles (10″). Do it again, tense up, tightly, clinch your teeth, pull the corners of your mouth back hard (5″) and relax, completely relaxed, warm and relaxed (10″). OK, good. Next do the neck and chin muscles. This is done by pulling in the chin very hard and tightening your neck muscles. Go ahead, tense them tightly, pull hard, very hard, (5″) and relax, no tension, let go completely, warm and relaxed (10″). Very good, you should be noticing that there is no tension when you let go and the relaxation flows through your muscles. Do your neck and chin again, pull in your chin. Tighten your neck muscles, hold tightly, (5″) and relax, feel the relaxation, very relaxed (10″). Now do the chest muscles and the upper back. These are hard to explain in words but you'll feel the muscles pull below your shoulders. OK, tense these muscles up, push your shoulders forward a bit, feel the muscles pull in your back (5″) and relax. Let them go all at once, completely. Warm and relaxed (10″). OK, do them again, tense up, feel the muscles pull in the back (5″) and relax. Completely relaxed, no tension, warm and relaxed (10″). Next do the muscles in the stomach–you tense these by making the stomach as hard as you can. Tense them up, make your stomach hard, pull in, very hard (5″) and relax. Relax completely (10″). OK, again . . . pull in the stomach, make it hard. Very hard, pull (5″) and relax, completely relaxed, warm and relaxed (10″). Good, now the leg muscles. Tighten up all of your leg muscles, tighten them up, very tight (5″) and relax. Relax completely, no tension (10″). Again, tense up your legs very tightly (5″) and relax. Completely relaxed, warm and relaxed (10″). That's good. The last muscles to do are those in your feet, and you can do these by curling your toes very tightly. Curl them tightly, very tightly, tightly (5″) and relax, relax completely, (10″). Again curl your toes, tightly, tightly (5″) and relax, completely relaxed, warm and relaxed, no tension (10″).

OK, now try to get everything relaxed at once, your whole body. Go through the muscles again as they are named and check to see it they have that same relaxed, limp feeling that they had when you first did them. See if you can get really relaxed–no tension. Start with your hands and the bottom part of your arms. If they are not totally relaxed, i.e., if you can feel some tension, tense them up slightly and relax them just as we did before (10″). Now the top of your arms and shoulders (10″), and then the upper part of the face—the eyes and forehead (10″). Now the lower part of the face—the mouth and jaw (10″). Pay attention to how relaxed your muscles are, chin (10″) and then the chest and upper back muscles, feel the relaxation (10″). Now the stomach muscles—no tension (10″). And next the legs, warm and relaxed (10″). Finally the feet and toes, completely relaxed, warm and relaxed, very relaxed (10″).

OK, fine, now concentrate on relaxing your whole body. Get your whole body as relaxed as you can. Each muscle group won't be named again, but if you still find some tension anywhere in any muscle, just tense that muscle up a little bit like before and then relax, relax completely, that warm feeling of no tension, completely relaxed, very relaxed (10″). Now take a deep breath, hold it (3″), let it out completely and relax, very relaxed, warm and relaxed (10″). Just stay relaxed, warm and relaxed. Go on relaxing for a few minutes. Allow subject to relax for 5 minutes. OK, now it's time to stop but you should do this slowly. Listen carefully. I will count to 4. On the count of "one" move your hands and arms all around to wake them up. On the count of "two" move your feet and legs all around. On "three" move your head and neck. On "four" open your eyes and sit up, moving your whole body around. OK. "One," move your hands and arms (5 sec.). "Two," move your feet and legs (5 sec). "Three," move your head and neck (5 sec). "Four," open your eyes, completely awake, sit up. Move all around a bit, then stand up and stretch.

APPENDIX J
How to Find out More about Both Allergy and Emotions (Bibliography)

Allergy

1. Allergy Foundation of America. *Allergy–Its Mysterious Causes and Treatment.* New York: Grosset & Dunlap, 1968.
2. Allergy Information Association, 3 Powburn Place, Weston 627, Ontario, Canada. (Everything you need to know; a very helpful organization.)
3. Bernack, Raymond J. *What is Allergy?* Springfield, Illinois: Charles C. Thomas, 1967.
4. Bottomly, Harold W. *Allergy–Its Treatment and Care.* Toronto: Longmans, 1968.
5. Environmental Health Association. *Manual for Those Sensitive to Foods, Drugs and Chemicals.* Washington, D.C., 1969.
6. Frazier, Claude A. *Parents' Guide to Allergy in Children.* Garden City, New York: Doubleday & Company, Inc., 1973.
7. Frazier, Claude A. *Coping With Food Allergy.* New York: Quadrangle, 1974.
8. Rapp, Doris J. *Allergies and Your Child.* New York: Holt, Rinehart & Winston, 1972.
9. Sammis, Florence E. *The Allergic Patient and His World.* Springfield, Illinois: Charles C. Thomas, 1953.
10. Superintendent of Documents, U.S. Government Printing Office, Washington, D.C. 20402.
11. Swartz, Harry F. *The Allergy Guide Book–A Practical Program of Prevention and Control.* New York: Unger, 1961, 1966.
12. Swartz, Harry F. *Allergy: What It Is and What To Do About It.* New York: Unger, 1949, 1966.

Emotions

1. Bonnell, John Southerland. *Do You Want to Be Healed?* New York: Harper & Row, 1968.

2. Chess, Stella; Thomas, Alexander; and Bush, Hervert G. *Your Child Is A Person.* New York: Viking Press, 1965.
3. Collins, Vincent P. *Me, Myself and You.* St. Meinrad, Indiana: Abbey Press, 1974.
4. Dennison, A. Dudley. *Shock It To Me, Doctor.* Grand Rapids, Michigan: Zondervan Publishing House, 1970.
5. Frazier, Claude A., ed. *Faith Healing.* New York: Thomas Nelson, Inc., 1973.
6. Ginott, Haim G. *Between Parent and Child.* New York: The MacMillan Company, 1965.
7. Hirt, Michael L. *Psychological and Allergic Aspects of Asthma.* Springfield, Illinois: Charles C. Thomas, 1962.
8. Holt, John. *How Children Fail.* New York: Pitman Publishing Co., 1964.
9. Jones, Arthur. *The Primeval Scream.* New York: Dell Publishing Co., 1970.
10. Maltz, Maxwell, *Psycho-Cybernetics.* New York: Prentice-Hall, Inc., 1960.
11. Parents' Magazine. *Guiding Your Child from 5 to 12.* New York: Parents' Magazine Enterprises, Inc., 1960.
12. Spock, Benjamin. *Raising Children in a Difficult Time.* New York: W. W. Norton & Company, Inc., 1974.
13. Wernick, Robert. *The Family.* New York: Time-Life Books, 1974.

APPENDIX K
Breathing for Home Use*

Your physician has given you this booklet on breathing training so that you can help yourself breathe more efficiently. This program is designed to train your abdominal muscles to assist your diaphragm in some of the work of breathing. As you get accustomed to this different kind of breathing, you can expect to feel better and be more active in daily life.

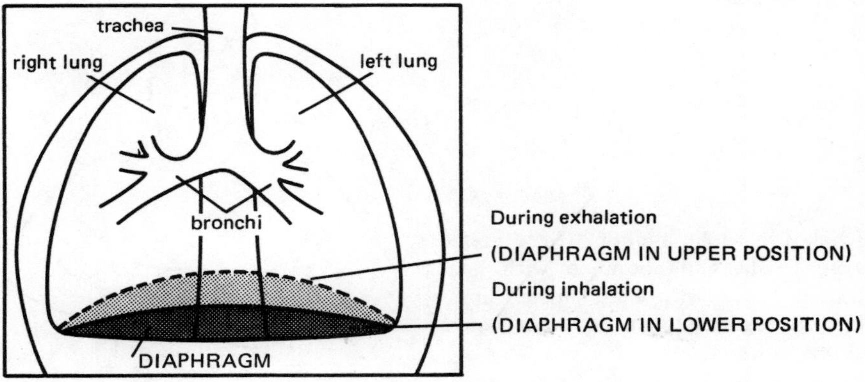

Your physician has checked the positions that are best for you at this time. The schedule of training may change as your new breathing techniques develop. Follow your physician's advice—and remember that the benefit you get from this program depends on the regularity and care with which you follow it daily.

Preparation

Breathing training is usually performed two to four times daily: on arising, before meals, during the late afternoon or just before retiring. The amount of time spent on each position will depend on your physician's directions.

*Breon Laboratories, Inc., 90 Park Avenue, New York, N.Y. 10016.

Before beginning your training, remove tight or restrictive clothing. Be sure your nasal passages are clear. If prescribed by your physician, inhale an aerosol medication according to his directions. This will relax and open the airways in your lungs, and help to loosen tenacious mucus so it can be more easily expectorated.

Most important, do not hurry your breathing training. Rest when necessary. Hold each position as long as instructed. And in all cases, begin your day with the BASIC MORNING POSITION as shown on page two of this booklet.

At-Home Breathing Training

Begin training sessions with aerosol medication as prescribed by your physician.

☐ BASIC MORNING POSITION

Sit erect on edge of bed or chair and place hands over lower ribs and upper abdomen as shown in Figure 1.
Keep shoulders down, elbows straight out, fingers rigid. Repeat 10 times, or as physician directs.

FIG. 1

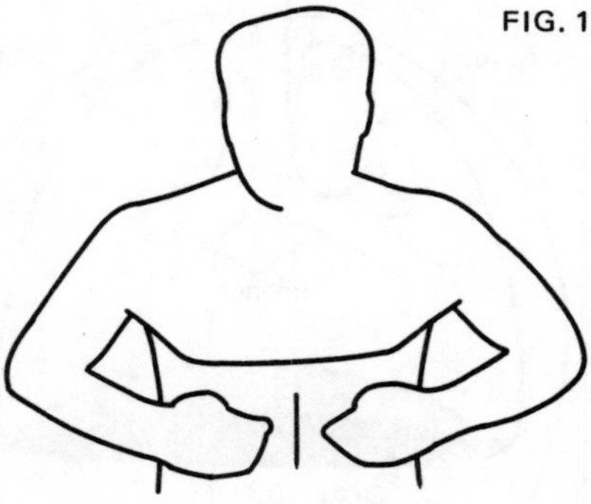

Fig. 1
EXHALE while applying firm pressure against ribs and abdomen with hands. Exhale slowly through pursed lips . . . lips held partly open as when you are about to whistle.

FIG. 2

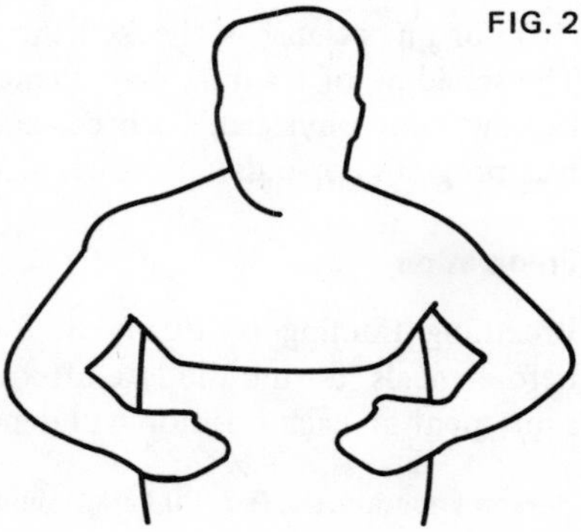

Fig. 2
INHALE after releasing pressure of hands slightly, but still applying effort against chest and abdomen. Cough gently to raise mucus.

☐ POSITION ONE

INHALE

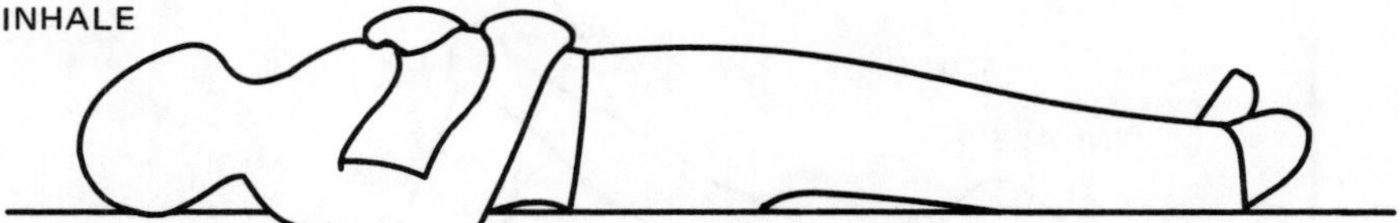

EXHALE

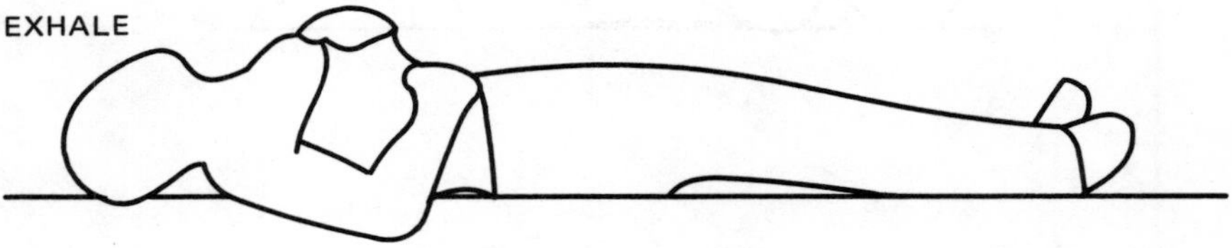

Lie flat on floor (*not* on bed) as shown, and rest left hand across chest, right hand on abdomen. Inhale deeply through nose, letting abdomen rise. Then breathe out through pursed lips, pressing inward and upward firmly on abdomen. Try to move the chest as little as possible, letting the abdomen move up and down as you inhale and exhale. As your physician directs, you may practice this way of breathing while sitting or standing. Repeat 6–8 times. Once you have developed this technique you should breathe in this manner even while walking.

☐ POSITION TWO

Lie flat on floor as shown, and rest left hand across chest, right hand on abdomen. Bend knees, keeping them together. Keep feet on floor, bringing thighs toward chest as far as possible. Inhale through nose, letting abdomen rise. Then breathe out through pursed lips, pressing inward and upward firmly on abdomen. Repeat 6–8 times, or as physician directs.

INHALE

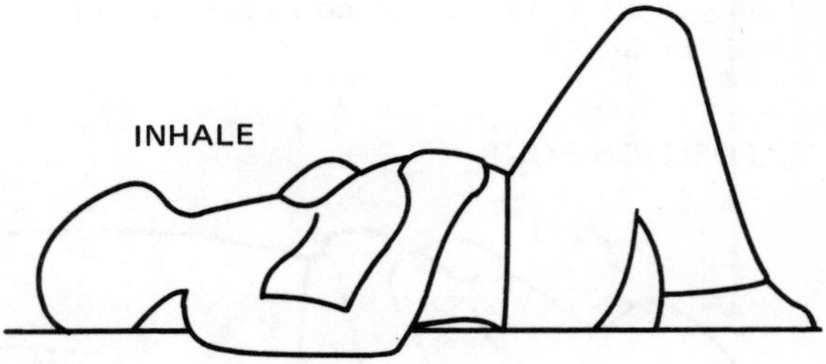

EXHALE

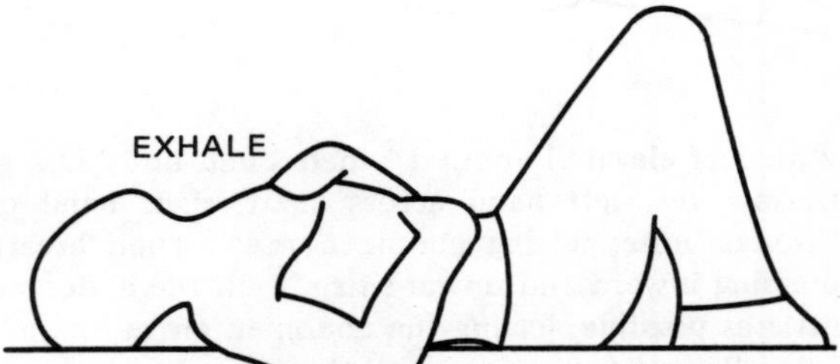

☐ POSITION THREE

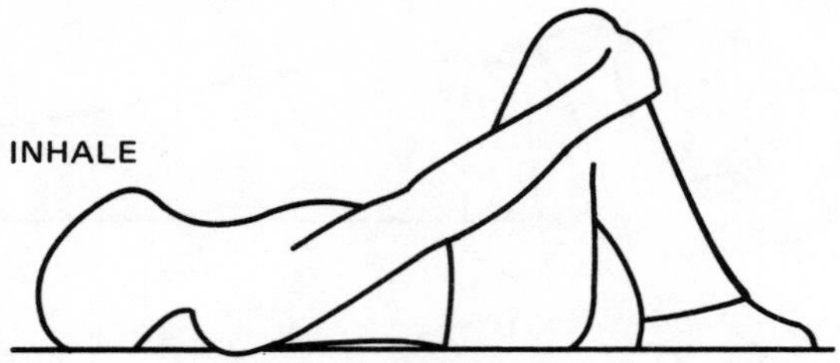

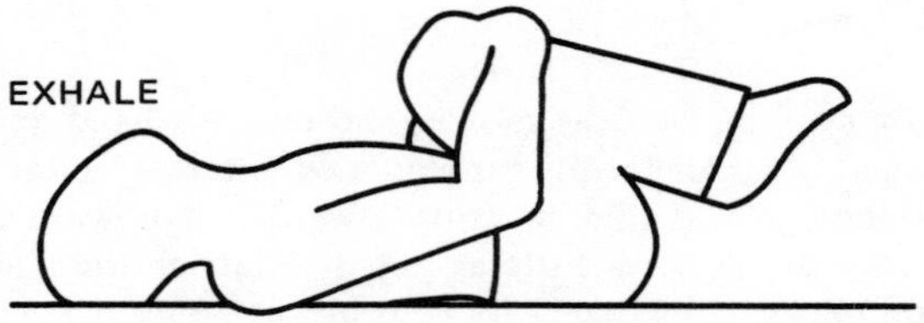

Lie flat on floor as shown, raise knees and lock arms around legs. Inhale through nose, letting abdomen rise. Lift feet from floor and exhale through pursed lips, pulling legs toward chest as far as possible with arms. Repeat 6–8 times, or as physician directs.

☐ POSITION FOUR

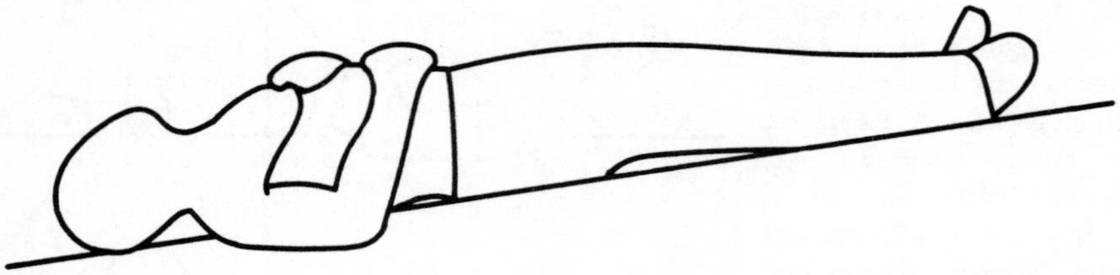

With feet elevated about 14 inches and body in a straight line as shown in illustration, rest left hand across chest, right hand on abdomen. Inhale deeply through nose, letting abdomen rise. Then breathe out through pursed lips, pressing inward and upward firmly on the abdomen. Try to move the chest as little as possible, letting the abdomen move up and down as you inhale and exhale. Repeat 6–8 times, or as physician directs.

☐ POSITION FIVE

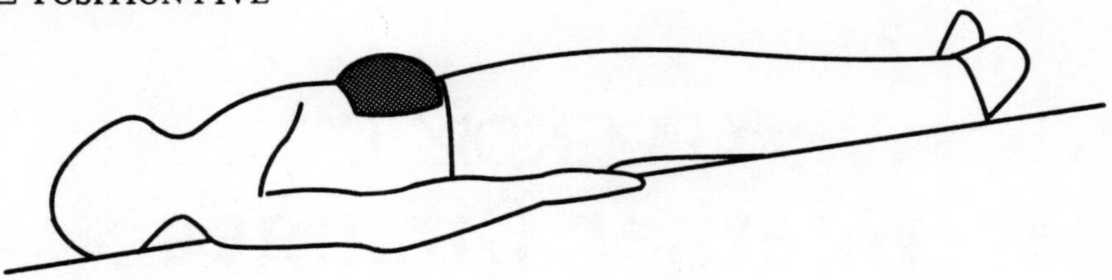

With feet elevated about 14 inches and body in a straight line as shown in illustration, place a five-pound weight on the abdomen. (Use rubber hot-water bottle, or cloth sack filled with sand.) Inhale deeply through nose, letting abdomen rise. Then breathe out through pursed lips. Physician may instruct you to gradually increase weight to 15 pounds. Repeat 6–8 times, or as physician directs.

APPENDIX L
Weather Changes and Temperature

Hay fever and asthma are WORSE at NIGHT AND in the EARLY MORNING hours because of COOL OR COLD AIR. Whenever weather permits, you should sleep with the bedroom windows closed, at other times with as few windows open as possible. A normal individual is not affected by weather and temperature changes, but the allergic individual is affected by slight drafts, and changes in temperature and humidity; drops in temperature with attending decreases in the moisture in the air most often are responsible for symptoms. It is, therefore, advisable to have the bedroom, at least, warm during the night. A temperature between 68° and 70°F., but NOT LOWER than 65°F., should be maintained throughout the night in the bedroom. Warm moist air is preferable to warm dry air. A wall thermometer is a great help toward regulating the temperature in the room. Of course, if the whole house can be kept at an even temperature, it is better than if only the bedroom is so kept. Humidity of the house should be approximately 40%.

Do not stay outdoors on cold, windy days. When you are outside during cold winter months dress warmly and wear either a hat or scarf. Avoid going outside for at least one hour after bathing during cold weather. Avoid going to bed with wet hair. Upon getting out of bed in the morning wear bedroom shoes. Avoid going barefooted in the summer. Avoid wearing wet bathing suit for prolonged period.

APPENDIX M
Social Readjustment Rating Scale*

Rank	*Life event*	*LCU (Life Change Unit) value*
1.	Death of spouse	100
2.	Divorce	73
3.	Marital separation	65
4.	Jail term	63
5.	Death of a close family member	63
6.	Personal injury or illness	53
7.	Marriage	50
8.	Fired from job	47
9.	Marital reconciliation	45
10.	Retirement	45
11.	Change in health of family member	44
12.	Pregnancy	40
13.	Sex difficulties	39
14.	Gain of new family member	39
15.	Business readjustment	39
16.	Change in financial state	38
17.	Death of close friend	37
18.	Change to different line of work	36
19.	Change in number of arguments with spouse	35
20.	Mortgage over $10,000	31
21.	Foreclosure of mortgage or loan	30
22.	Change in responsibilities at work	29
23.	Son or daughter leaving home	29
24.	Trouble with in-laws	29

*Thomas H. Holmes and Richard Rahe.

Rank	*Life event*	*LCU (Life Change Unit) value*
25.	Outstanding personal achievement	28
26.	Wife begins or stops work	26
27.	Begin or end school	26
28.	Change in living conditions	25
29.	Revision of personal habits	24
30.	Trouble with boss	23
31.	Change in work hours or conditions	20
32.	Change in residence	20
33.	Change in schools	20
34.	Change in recreation	19
35.	Change in church activities	19
36.	Change in social activities	18
37.	Mortgage or loan less than $10,000	17
38.	Change in sleeping habits	16
39.	Change in number of family get-togethers	15
40.	Change in eating habits	15
41.	Vacation	13
42.	Christmas	12
43.	Minor violations of the law	11

INDEX

INDEX